Shatter the Yoyo

A Definitive Guide to Losing Weight and Gaining Self Control While Ending Your Dependence on Diets

DR. CANDICE SETI, PSY. D

Shatter the Yoyo

DISCLAIMER: The information contained in this book is for informational purposes only. It is not a substitute for the advice and care of healthcare professionals. Further, this book is not a medical manual. It is an account of one approach to weight management. The author, editor, and publisher expressly disclaim responsibility for any adverse effects that might result from using or applying the information contained in this book.

None of the individuals involved in writing, editing, producing, or publishing this book are rendering professional services to the individual reader. Although efforts have been made to ensure the accuracy of all information contained in this book, the author(s), editors, publishers, and printers do not assume responsibility for any errors that inadvertently have been included.

Neither the author nor the publisher is engaged in rendering professional advice or services to the individual reader. The ideas, procedures, and suggestions contained in this book are not intended as a substitute for consulting with your healthcare professionals. All matters regarding your health require medical supervision. Neither the author nor the publisher shall be liable or responsible for any loss or damage allegedly arising from any information or suggestion in this book.

All images in this book are either owned by the author or labeled "free to reuse" or are "royalty-free stock photos."

Names of individuals in this book have been changed.

ISBN: 978-1-946978-28-8

Dedication

For Matt

Thank you for your limitless support and belief
in me and for your willingness to always be my
first guinea pig!

Contents

Section 1—Setting the Stage..ix

Chapter 1—What This Program Is and Isn't............................1

Chapter 2—Yoyo Dieting in a Nutshell
(and It Ain't Pretty) 5

Chapter 3—Keys to Success—Change Your Focus,
Change Your Thoughts, Change Your Life......................11

Chapter 4—The Dirt on Dieting.....................................17

Chapter 5—It's Not All in Your Head: How Biology
Keeps the Yoyo Going...23

Section 2—Change Your Focus..................................41

Chapter 6—Are You Focusing on the Right Things? 43

Chapter 7—Focusing on the Goals of Your Goals 49

Chapter 8—From Restriction to Permission (Yes, Ice
Cream Can Really Be a Regular Part of Your Life).......57

Chapter 9—Saying Goodbye to Our Diet Language 67

Section 3—Change Your Thoughts 75

Chapter 10—Understanding Automatic Thoughts.............77

Chapter 11—Cognitive Distortions: Automatic
Thoughts Gone Wrong...81

Chapter 12—Cognitive Distortions Versus Reasonable
Responses 93

Chapter 13—Power Thoughts: Helping to Keep
Cognitive Distortions at Bay 99

Section 4—Change Your Life 107

Chapter 14—The Power of Habits.............................109

Chapter 15—Know Thy Enemy: Identifying Your
Danger Zones...115

Chapter 16—Actions Plans: Taking the Danger Out
of Danger Zones...141

Section 5—Stacking the Odds in Your Favor 165

Chapter 17—The Power of Self-Care.........................167

Chapter 18—Adding to Your "No More Yoyo Dieting"
Toolbox..181

Chapter 19—Words of Wisdom When the Going
Gets Tough..189

Section 6—Trouble Shooting 197

Chapter 20—Getting Back on Track When It Feels
Like It's All Falling Apart.............................199

Chapter 21—What to Do When You're Getting Better
Slowly, But You Want to Lose Weight Fast.....207

Chapter 22—A Body Image Gone Wrong . . .
Then Radical Acceptance 213

Section 7—Putting It All Together 215

Chapter 23—A Week in the Life of a (Former)
Yoyo Dieter, Before and After This Program....217

Chapter 24—Next Steps...225

Section 8—Conclusion 233

Acknowledgements 237

About the Author...239

Setting the Stage

CHAPTER 1

What This Program Is and Isn't

"When I let go of what I am,
I become what I might be."

—LAO TZU

Welcome to Shatter the Yoyo! You are about to embark on a journey that has the potential to be life changing and to help you achieve your food, weight, and shape goals. I've written this book as a psychologist, a nutrition coach, and a personal trainer but also as a reformed yoyo dieter. In other words, I bring a lot of expertise and a lot of real-world experience to this program. And that is why I am confident that this program can help yoyo dieters finally free themselves from the diet/binge cycle that leads to so much unhappiness for so many people.

Before getting into the substance of the program, it's important to understand what this program is and isn't. This program is a collection of tools (skills) that I have gathered together for the express purpose of helping you end the cycle of weight loss and weight gain that can steal vast amounts of your life and leave you feeling ashamed and defeated.

This program reflects years of education, clinical experience, and my own firsthand knowledge of what it takes to (re)learn how to listen to your body and lose weight **without** dieting. My approach combines cognitive behavioral therapy, self-care, and paying close attention to biological factors, like sleep and hydration, into a single program that you can work through at your own pace.

This book is also quite interactive. Most chapters will have you engaging in brainstorming activities or creating action plans. As such, most chapters will include worksheets. (Look for the green check mark to let you know you have an assignment!) If you are a "pen and paper" kind of person, you can write directly in the book or make photocopies. If you prefer to work on your computer or tablet, you can download all the worksheets in one workbook directly from www.ShatterTheYoyoWorkbook.com.

In addition, if you decide you want to take your work in this area even further, I do offer a full, online, weight-loss and weight-management program that will go significantly more in-depth. It covers many additional areas that I will discuss later in the book. If you want to check that out, feel free to visit www.ShatterTheYoyo.com.

I can't promise the fast results that you might get from yet another diet, but I can tell you that this approach is what finally allowed me to lose weight and keep it off. It's also what has given me back the peace of mind about food and weight that I had before I took a wrong turn and ended up on that dead-end street known as yoyo dieting.

The tools I introduce in this manual might also prove useful for issues outside of weight management. For example, improving your sleep might improve your mood. Making sure you stay hydrated might help keep up your energy levels throughout the day. But, even though this program might offer benefits outside of its weight management focus, it was not designed to do so. For example, mood disorders, attention deficit hyperactivity disorder (ADHD), obsessive-compulsive disorder (OCD), or trauma-related symptoms are not the focus of this manual. If you need to manage these (or other) symptoms at the same time as you are working on achieving weight management success, please make sure you get the appropriate professional support.

This program cannot offer all that you need. Further, this program is much more likely to be successful if other medical conditions, be they psychological and/or physical, are getting the attention they deserve. So, make sure to let your healthcare professionals know that you are following this program. They might be able to offer suggestions that reinforce the work you are doing or at least offer treatment that takes into the account the steps outlined in this book.

The bottom line is that this program is designed to help you finally manage your weight successfully, a goal that is so elusive for so many. It wouldn't surprise me if other parts of your life also got better! (But don't count on this program to be a panacea!) Other problems might need other solutions. Along those lines, it is important to be clear that this book does not replace medical care by the appropriate professionals.

Phew, now that we have that out of the way, let's look at the program.

CHAPTER 2

Yoyo Dieting in a Nutshell (and It Ain't Pretty)

"If you do what you've always done, you'll get what you've always gotten."

—TONY ROBBINS

If you are reading this book, chances are really good you've been on a diet (or 20!) before. Chances are also really good that you've lost weight on that diet. And last, chances are also really good that you've gained back the weight you lost. You are not alone (to put it mildly)! The data on the long-term success of diets is startling, especially when you realize that only about 2 percent of people who go on diets are able to lose weight **and** successfully keep it off. You'd assume that this fact alone would have people thinking twice about going on a diet. I mean with a failure rate of 98 percent, who really wants to play those odds?

Well, apparently a lot of people. Dieting is a multi-billion-dollar business in the United States alone. Diet books are regularly on the best-seller list, and there is no end to diet-related headlines jumping out from magazines and tabloid television shows. So, why are there so many diets out there and why do so many people subscribe to them, despite the gloomy failure rate? The short answer? Well, it looks easy. Most diets are well-packaged, easy-to-follow, clear cut, and designed to show results quickly. And who doesn't want immediate results? Naturally, we buy into a well-packaged diet program, jump onboard, and LOVE it, because we successfully lose weight (at first). That's the goal, right?

The problem is that it is a short-term result, when what we are really looking for is long -term success. Even when you start to realize that diets don't seem to work the way you had hoped, you are drawn in by the quick results. You want instant success, instant satisfaction—or as close to instant as you can get. So, you are thrilled with your success, and you stay on the diet for as long as you can stand it. Then what? Slowly, but steadily, you gain that weight back. And you know what happens when you realize you've gained it back? You jump right back on that diet that didn't give you any long-term success!

It's crazy when you stand back and think about it (even though millions of us fall victim to the same pattern)! But if you just focus on the days and weeks (instead of months and years) in front of us, it starts to make sense. We associate that diet with being successful, because the last time we did it, we lost weight, felt great, and loved it! The other problem is that a lot of us don't know what else to do. Sure, we have played enough versions of the dieting game to know that we're going to end up bitterly disappointed eventually. But what else are we supposed to do? Give up and not even try?

The combination of short-term success and no apparent alternative takes us right back to dieting. This time, it's going to work, right? Maybe for a few weeks or months. Maybe even longer for a few people. But then the weight starts to return, uninvited and unwanted. Weight-loss success isn't ours after all. And on and on it goes. This is the classic yoyo dieting phenomenon.

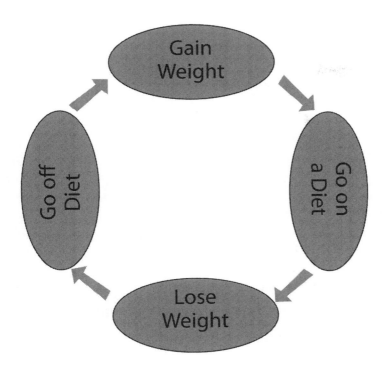

And this phenomenon results in big problems for most dieters. Let's take a moment to look at just how big this problem really is:

- ➤ 98 percent of diets fail (yes, 98 percent!), and most people will regain any weight lost within one year.
- ➤ 91 percent of women have attempted to control their weight through dieting, and about 50 percent of women are on a diet at any given point in time.
- ➤ The obesity industry accounts for 3 percent of the overall US economy—that's more than $315 billion a year!
- ➤ Americans spend more money on dieting than any other country in the world.

> ➤ The incidence of childhood obesity has tripled since the 1980s.
> ➤ 35 percent of dieters become "addicted" to dieting—aka yoyo dieters.

So, what does this mean for you? Is it really such a big deal if you keep yoyo dieting? After all, diets do help you lose weight, so what if you have to do it over and over again? You can just keep going back to it, right? And, maybe the latest dieting fad is the one that will really work for you this time. Well, anything is possible. But here's the real problem. Statistics tell us that the vast majority of people will regain the weight they lost, and this yoyo dieting has a massive dark side! There are several different reasons for this, some well-known, some less so. Either way, it's important that we all have our eyes open when it comes to the problems that can be triggered by yoyo dieting:

> ➤ Yoyo dieting has a major impact on your self-perception and your view of your body. Repeated yoyo dieting can leave you with extremely negative feelings toward your body.
> ➤ Frequent yoyo dieting can lead to chronic sadness. This is partly due to the negative self-concept that develops and partly due to the emotional instability that is caused by weight that goes down, then up, then down, and then up again.
> ➤ Yoyo dieting can leave you feeling dependent and out of control. You can feel trapped, as if you have no other option than to be constantly on or off a diet.
> ➤ Yoyo dieting results in an incredibly unhealthy relationship with food. This relationship often leads to viewing food as either being all "bad" or all "good." It can feel like food

has total control over your behavior and that you are "less than" other people who are slim and healthy.

➤ Yoyo dieting can wreak havoc on your metabolism. When you lose weight, your metabolism can drop, particularly if you have lost weight quickly. This is your body's normal response to the "famine" you have created by going on a diet. But when the inevitable happens and you fall off the diet and begin to eat more (sometimes a lot more!), your metabolism doesn't bounce back as quickly. That's why the weight you lost is much easier to regain and even harder to lose again. This cycle only gets worse and worse the longer you continue to be an on-again, off-again dieter.

➤ Yoyo dieting can cause hormonal changes that make it harder to lose weight. The hormones that manage stress and hunger can end up out of whack from frequent dieting. This can make your appetite voracious and convinces your body to hold onto fat, just in case another "famine" (that is, a diet) is coming around again.

➤ Frequent yoyo dieting can encourage the build-up of visceral fat in the mid-section. Sometimes carrying a lot of your extra weight around your mid-section/abdomen is a sign that visceral fat is starting to collect. Because visceral fat is associated with medical conditions like angina, heart disease, stroke, and heart attacks, it is something you definitely want to control. With yoyo dieting, you think you are putting time and energy into getting healthier only to end up less healthy than when you started. That sounds like a deal that you're better off refusing!

That's quite a list, huh? Given all this, it should be clear that the time to change this pattern is NOW! Not next year, next month, or even next week. The longer you wait, the harder it will be. That being said, even if have spent decades as a yoyo dieter, it is still possible to get off that train (which is headed to nowhere good, even as I write this)! Sure, your habits might be a bit harder to break, but with enough effort, even those of you who have been diehard weight-loss, weight-gain cyclers for years can benefit from this program.

In other words, whether you've been on one diet or so many you can't even keep track, hope is not lost. You can gain control without feeling dependent on a structured diet program. You can manage your weight without dieting. You can stop hyperfocusing on calories, points, or macros. You can stop the yoyo dieting cycle for good. You can be free.

CHAPTER 3

Keys to Success—Change Your Focus, Change Your Thoughts, Change Your Life

"When it becomes more difficult to suffer than to change . . . you will change."

—ROBERT ANTHONY

In this book, you will learn various aspects of my Shatter the Yoyo program. Using the techniques I will be introducing, you will finally be able to manage your weight without dieting. The model below is an overview of the program that will be unfolding in the coming pages.

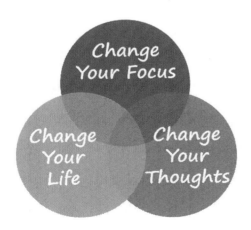

As you can see, the program is based on three main concepts—changing your focus, changing your thoughts, and changing your life. Let me briefly introduce each of these program components.

Step 1: We start with changing your focus. This step is about challenging the beliefs and behaviors that you cling to because of all the previous dieting. People don't always realize how ingrained diet concepts become over time. It's important to recognize and change this part of your psyche. If you don't, your dieting mindset can keep you stuck and stop you from developing the thoughts and behaviors that are so important for breaking free of the weight gain–weight-loss yoyo.

Step 2: We will be working on changing your thoughts. You might not realize just how your every day, "regular" thoughts are impacting your relationship with food and your ability to lose weight and keep it off. In fact, most people are blissfully unaware of the impact their thinking has on many different aspects of their life. But to truly gain control and break out of the yoyo dieting world for good, you need to become aware of your thoughts. Once you have this awareness, you will be able to replace some of your old ways of thinking with new, more effective thoughts. And by effective, I mean thoughts that won't stand in the way of weight loss. Instead these new, productive thoughts will help you develop a relaxed, peaceful relationship with food **and** let go of the extra weight that dieting invited into your life.

Step 3: We help you understand that changing the way you live your life is an important part of your future. What does that mean? This is where you will be really digging into your lifestyle. I will introduce the skills you need to recognize the behavioral patterns that set you up for failure, make success difficult, or leave you without options. Sometimes the simplest changes to the environment can have the biggest impact. You won't really know what changes you need to make until you examine your lifestyle and determine where your trouble spots are. Once you do that, you can restructure and create new, healthy, more adaptive patterns for yourself that don't require so much effort!

If you find at the end of this book that you want to keep working on developing skills that will allow you to successfully manage your weight, I offer a more in-depth Shatter the Yoyo program online. The online program not only expands on the information provided in this book, it also covers other aspects of weight management, including mindful eating, food prep, kitchen setup, meal time setup, and stress management.

I offer this additional program because I truly believe that the more skills and tools you have, the more equipped you are to ditch yoyo dieting for good and live your life as the best possible version of you. Not only does the online program leave you even more prepared to make the changes necessary to finally (!) enjoy successful weight management, it also comes with direct Skype coaching sessions with me! I can't wait to help each and every one of you uncover your body's natural ability to manage its weight and your ability to eat without anxiety or binge-induced guilt.

My Story

But why should you listen to me about any of this? Really who am I to talk? Many people look at me and think, "She doesn't have a weight problem . . . what does she know about it? How can she relate?"

Well, the truth is, I've been there. Growing up I was a beanpole—skin and bones. I could eat anything, anytime, without impact. A half-gallon of ice cream, sure. An entire pizza, no problem. Of course, I didn't really appreciate how lucky I was until the end of high school. That's when I noticed that other girls had issues with weight and often talked about calories, and dieting—things I knew nothing about. Well, I maintained my ignorance in those areas until I was about 24 years old.

That was when things started to change. I didn't really notice it at first. Yes, I was buying clothes in a bigger size, but I didn't really give it a second thought. As far as I was concerned, I was filling out. That didn't seem to be such a problem. That is until I really stopped and took a good, long look at myself. I found I no longer liked what I saw when I looked in the mirror. I no longer felt comfortable in my skin. The biggest problem with this was that I HAD ABSOLUTELY NO IDEA what to do about it! I had never paid attention to health, ingredients, calories, ANYTHING! I just ate. A lot.

So, naturally, I went on one of the diets I saw advertised on TV. Everyone loses weight on those diets, and besides, they were so easy, right? I went in every week, weighed in, and picked up my food. And I lost weight—40 pounds, when all was said and done. I was thrilled! I felt great. I was proud of my success and was happy in my skin again. So, of course, I stopped the diet.

I'm fairly sure you can guess what happened to me during the next year. Yep, you guessed it! I started to gain it all back. When it was less than 10 pounds of regain, I wasn't so concerned, but as more and more of the weight I had so recently lost came back, well, I was frustrated! As you might expect, my natural reaction was to decide to go back on the diet. I mean it worked before! Shouldn't I just do it again? Well I did—three more times. Until I finally said, "What the ???"

This was my magic moment—the moment when everything changed for me. It just clicked in my head that it didn't make sense. Was I going to have to keep going back on this diet every six months for the rest of my life? Was I stuck going back and forth with my weight? Wasn't there any long-term solution? Did I really have to live like this?

So, I decided to do something different. Do things my own way— even though I wasn't quite sure what that meant. ;-) Thanks to the diet program, I knew really well how to count calories and that whole game. What I knew nothing about was my relationship with food. I didn't know how I used food, why I ate when I did, how I made the food decisions I made, or what made my body feel good. So, being a psychologist, I decided to become my own clinical study. I decided to spend time examining my relationship with food and my body until I could finally answer all the questions I had about managing my weight.

To say I learned a lot in this process is the understatement of the century. I had no idea how reliant I was on food; to make me feel better, to cure my boredom, and to give me energy. I had no idea that the most common reasons I ate were because I was bored or because food just happened to be nearby and available. And I REALLY had no idea what foods made my body feel good. It was almost as if actual physical hunger didn't even fit into the equation when it came to my eating. Dieting had made me lose sight of what my body needed and when it needed it. Instead, dieting had replaced my body's own wisdom with rules and regulations that promised to make weight loss "easy" but instead made weight gain even easier!

So, after learning all this about myself, through a lot of trial and error, I was able to make changes. Changes to my thinking, changes to my behavior, and changes to my lifestyle. Changes that I have easily kept up since—for more than a decade. Once that happened, I never went on a diet again. And I never worried about my weight again. I felt good, I was in great shape, and more important, I was happy.

The process was so eye-opening for me that I decided to devote my life to sharing it with others. I knew I wanted to continue my practice as a psychologist, but I wanted to tweak it to focus on weight management and the relationship people have with food. I wanted to help others the way I'd helped myself and give them the same freedom that I had attained. I went back to school and got certified as a nutrition coach and a personal trainer so that I could truly focus on the whole picture with my clients. And I have loved every minute of it!

So, there you have it—I *can* relate. Not only have I been right where you are, but I have firsthand experience of getting out of the trap of weight loss and weight (re)gain by using this program. I know that this program works; not because I read about it in some scientific journal or studied it in some class. I know that this program works, because it's what I used to finally "shatter the yoyo!"

CHAPTER 4
The Dirt on Dieting

"The definition of insanity is doing the same thing over and over and expecting different results."

—ATTRIBUTED TO ALBERT EINSTEIN

Dieting is nothing new. In fact, the first known diet dates all the way back to 1724! In 1863, a popular diet emerged that really laid the groundwork for the diets we have today. For as many years as diets have been around, there are even more types of diets—many of which are just variants of the same thing. What all diets have in common is some type of restriction—low fat, low carb, low dairy, low sodium, gluten free, vegetarian, no soy, high fat, high protein, raw, and on it goes. If there's something to restrict, chances are there's a diet that's been built around it!

The fact that there are SO many different diets out there is proof of a few points.

(1) There has yet to be a diet that works in the long term. (That's why people keep inventing new diets!)

(2) There is no one-size-fits-all approach to weight loss.

(3) There are a lot of people in the business of selling diets— because they do work. Work to make money, that is.

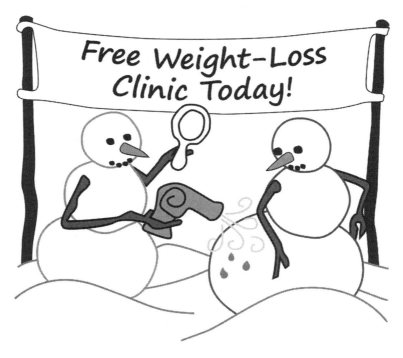

For many of the past decades, especially the 1980s and 1990s, there have been a seemingly endless supply of fad diets. Remember when low fat was all the rage and every food company on the planet was trying to make a low-fat line of products? This was also about the time when the media was starting to have power over our thinking—via television commercials, print ads, radio ads, billboards, etc. Fad diets were everywhere, and everything was about being skinny, no matter what the cost. Diet pills were being taken in abundance—Dexatrim, Ephedra, fen-phen, Metabolife, TrimSpa, etc. They were all basically variants of stimulants or amphetamines and all had the potential to cause severe side effects. But the diet mentality was officially engrained in us as a culture. It was not about health or wellness—it was about weight loss. Period.

While the focus on dieting might still be rampant in our culture, I am a little bit hopeful that the tides are turning. It seems to me that, as a culture, we are slowly learning to focus on health rather than the dieting mentality. Unfortunately, it took a lot of negative statistics to bring that about. Perhaps the biggest factor has been the obesity epidemic. In case you missed it, we have a major obesity epidemic in this country that seemed to begin in the mid-1990s. Here are some important facts about that epidemic:

➢ More than 2/3 of adults are considered overweight; 1/3 of US adults are obese.

➢ More than 1 in 20 adults are considered extremely obese.

➢ 74 percent of adult men are overweight or obese.

➢ More than 1/3 of children and adolescents are overweight or obese.

➢ Obesity-related conditions are among the leading causes of death in the United States.

➢ The annual medical cost of obesity in the United States is more than $147 billion.

There is no question that obesity is a huge issue in the United States. With increased awareness of obesity and its health impacts (for example, type 2 diabetes, metabolic syndrome, osteoarthritis) has come a renewed focus on health and well-being. People seem to be aware of health now more than ever. Organic and whole food-based products are getting easier to find in the local grocery store. People are focused on exercise as a means of developing strength instead of simply burning calories. (You've probably heard the phrase "strong is the new skinny.") And people are choosing to live more active lifestyles by walking or biking, using stand-up desks, and engaging in other activities. This is promising evidence of good changes to come!

But the obesity epidemic also brings the potential for more and more people to become yoyo dieters. When it comes to weight loss, it seems that a lot of people are more "rabbit" than "hare," which makes the "lose weight fast" promise of fad diets hard to resist. What makes it even harder to resist is that the downside of dieting isn't nearly as well publicized or discussed as the dieting "success stories" that dominate television, magazines, and social media. Without an understanding of the damage that dieting can cause for some people, it isn't all that difficult to recruit another generation of yoyo dieters. My hope is that this program will be able to catch people early in their dieting efforts and help them transition from a focus on restriction to a focus on health and wellness.

Time for Change

I believe that this renewed focus on health and wellness is something that can continue to grow. This program has been designed to contribute to the positive changes happening in the field of weight management. It has also been designed to help anyone and everyone who wants to learn how to truly change their relationships with food. It is my mission to help as many people as possible to escape the world of yoyo dieting and spare them years of frustration and self-hatred.

Now, here you are, reading this book. I'm going to guess that is because several of the following are true:

- ✓ You feel dependent on diets to manage your weight.
- ✓ Your weight is always fluctuating.
- ✓ You think in terms of points, calories, or macros.
- ✓ You think about food. A LOT!
- ✓ You have lots of different-sized clothes in your closet.

✓ You have a history of restricting foods.

✓ You get anxious when you are expected to go out to eat with other people.

✓ Your weight has continued to go up, despite all the effort you put into dieting.

✓ The scale gives you anxiety, yet you use it regularly.

✓ You are sick of people commenting on your weight.

Any of these sound like you? I'm also going to guess that several of the following are things you want to achieve:

✓ Maintaining your weight on your own with minimal effort.

✓ Ending your weight fluctuations.

✓ Putting an end to the binge eating that often follows "successful" diets.

✓ No longer being obsessed with food and what you should or should not be eating.

✓ Feeling like you have self-control.

✓ Having a closet full of clothes, all of which fit.

✓ Enjoying eating.

✓ Not being anxious about eating in public or with friends.

✓ Feeling good in your body and your clothes.

✓ Having people see YOU, instead of your frequent weight gains and losses.

Here's the thing—the old way has been done. You've tried the diets. You've tried the fads. They didn't work or you wouldn't be reading this. The good news is there's a different way to approach weight management. A way that might take some effort to learn but which can continue to work for the rest of your life.

If you take control, follow this program, and commit to the behavioral and lifestyle changes needed to free yourself from dieting, great things can happen. It's up to you to decide whether you are ready to finally give up the yoyo dieting merry-go-round and be free of food and weight obsessions once and for all!

Chapter 5

It's Not All in Your Head: How Biology Keeps the Yoyo Going

"Your body is precious. It is your vehicle for awakening. Treat it with care."

—BUDDHA

Dieting Yourself (Super) Hungry

Make no mistake, emotions and distorted thinking can play a big part in yoyo dieting. They can be part of the reason you've been stuck going on and off diets for so many years. And this program is giving you the tools to take away the power these feelings and thoughts have had over you (and your weight)! But it's also good to know that it isn't ALL in your head. Sometimes when you can't think of anything but how many cookies you're going to eat as soon as you get home, it's biology leading the way. How and why is that even possible?

First, how is it that your body can "make you" eat a sleeve of Oreos even when you really, really don't want to regain all the weight you lost during the past two weeks, two months, or two years? Well, that's the power of hormones, of neurotransmitters (the chemicals in your brain) and of your body's "famine" response. Now, used well, these things are really, really important for keeping you healthy (and alive, for that matter). So, we actually like the chemicals coursing through our veins that work diligently to keep our blood sugar even, our mood level, and our metabolism ticking away. But all the good work they do can go awry when you're "starving" yourself during the day (okay, not literally starving, but restricting your food so much that you're darn hungry).

When faced with your own homemade famine (that is, this week's diet), hormones (such as leptin, ghrelin, insulin, and cortisol) can contribute to some appetite havoc. **Ghrelin** (the hormone responsible for making your stomach "growl" with hunger) gets higher when you are dieting—suddenly your "average" appetite has become the appetite of a bear. **Cortisol**, a literal life saver when facing acute stress, can join ghrelin in the "I could eat everything in the house" department when around for too long and/or in greater than normal amounts. Why would cortisol, a stress hormone, go up with dieting? Well, because yoyo dieting isn't exactly a walk in the park. And when it has been ongoing for years, it becomes a chronic stressor. **Leptin** and **insulin** are tied in with ghrelin and cortisol and can also make normal hunger seem like a distant memory. When no longer present at the right time or in the right amount, all four of these hormones can gang up on your metabolism, leaving it slow as molasses so that you gain weight even when you're not eating that much. (Hence the far too familiar rebound weight gain that closely follows a bout of "successful"—although apparently not so successful—dieting.)

But why? Why would your own body chemicals lead you so far away from the path to healthy weight management? You can thank your ancestors for that. Evolution left them with some finely honed systems, designed to help hold on to weight when famine arrived. It's far easier to survive a shortage of food if your body can slow down its use of calories and hold on to as much fat as possible. Just like it's wise to hold on to your money when cash is in short supply, your body knows that it's a really good idea to hold on to its calories when food is in short supply. Genius. But only if the famine is the real deal.

If the "famine" is, in fact, another episode of dieting, then the metabolism slows, even though there is no real shortage of food. And then, there you are, "breaking" the diet and eating every chocolate bar, hamburger, and pint of ice cream in sight. And, of course, you're doing that at the same time that your metabolism thinks it's doing you a favor by slowing down to a grinding halt. Presto, you've gained 10 pounds in two weeks.

This also explains why weight loss is often quicker at the start of a diet and then plateaus to nearly nothing, even if you're sticking firmly to the diet. What worked in week 1 of the diet, just isn't working in week 10, because your metabolism has slowed itself down. Post-diet weight gain and diets that seem to stop working for no apparent reason are the bane of all dieters. And they can certainly trigger a whole host of emotions and distorted thinking: "I'm a failure," "I have no willpower," "I'm pathetic," and "I'm never going to get out of this!"

If you simply aren't aware of the biology of dieting, it's easy to start blaming yourself for the diet "failure," rather than recognizing that the appetite and metabolism changes you are experiencing are entirely predictable. They are also the result of human biology, the same biology that would have kept you alive when facing a famine ten thousand years ago. It is also the biology that is keeping you far heavier than you want in the here and now.

Sleep

Freeing yourself from yoyo dieting means keeping biology on your side, not working against you. And that means making choices that bring out the best in your body chemistry (for example, hormones and neurotransmitters), not the worst. Sleep is a vital part of any weight-loss program and every healthy lifestyle. There is extensive data showing that sleep is integral to health. Sleep deprivation, fragmented sleep, or irregular sleep patterns (think shift work) have been linked to risk of weight gain, increased snacking, increased cravings, lower metabolism, lower willpower around junk food, increased stress levels, and less fat burning.

That is a significant list that clearly shows the connection between poor sleep and weight issues. A lot of the relationship between sleep and weight can be explained by the way sleep impacts hormone regulation. Remember the hormones that went awry in response to dieting? Disturbed sleep has its own impact on these powerful chemicals. Just take a gander at this list:

- **Ghrelin:** Remember, ghrelin is a hormone produced in the body that stimulates appetite. Because you don't require a tremendous amount of energy during sleep, ghrelin levels decrease significantly during slumber. This means if you are not sleeping well, your ghrelin levels don't decrease as much as they should, and your body thinks it's hungry when it's actually well nourished. Higher than normal ghrelin levels will also cause your body to stop burning calories in response to this perceived hunger! Double whammy!

- **Leptin:** Leptin is a hormone that functions opposite to ghrelin—it controls hunger and the feeling of satiety that comes from eating right and eating enough. Additionally, leptin is believed to be responsible for managing the way your body stores fat. As opposed to ghrelin, leptin levels increase during sleep so your brain knows it's satiated and doesn't having to worry about eating for a while. Of course, when you don't sleep enough, your leptin levels don't increase enough and, again, your brain thinks it needs food when it doesn't. Eventually, this can create constant hunger and a slow metabolism.

- **Insulin:** Insulin is a hormone that regulates blood glucose levels. Not getting enough ZZZs can cause insulin levels to rise by making your fat cells less sensitive to insulin. This impairs your body's ability to burn fat in addition to raising your risk for diabetes and cardiovascular diseases.

- **Cortisol:** Cortisol is one of the body's stress hormones, and when you're sleep deprived, cortisol impacts weight much like insulin does. Cortisol levels naturally decrease in the evening to prepare the body for sleep. However, in individuals who are sleep deprived, this process is impaired, and they maintain higher cortisol levels. Eventually, this can lead to insulin resistance, which increases your risk of type 2 diabetes. Cortisol is also an appetite stimulant, but it doesn't just leave us wanting to eat anything. Cortisol particularly increases our interest in high-sugar, high-fat foods. Watch out doughnuts, here we come!

Knowing all that we do about the connection between sleep and weight management, one of the first steps you should take in this program is ensuring you are getting the right quantity and quality of sleep. (Eight hours of tossing and turning just won't cut it.) Need some tips? Use this list to start building sleep habits that will leave you feeling well rested, energized, and without an appetite or metabolism gone wrong:

➤ Exercise at least 30 minutes/day (although not too close to bedtime, as increased body temperature can interfere with sleep onset). Exercise is known to improve sleep quality.

➤ Make your sleeping environment as dark as possible. Consider getting blackout curtains or using an eye mask. Making it dark includes not having a digital clock staring at you all night and not having a cell phone at your bedside that lights up every time a friend posts on social media. Turn the digital clock toward the wall, turn your cell phone off (if you can. If you can't, at least find a strategic, sleep-preserving location for it).

➤ Avoid alcohol, caffeine, and tobacco near bedtime.

➤ Keep the temperature of your bedroom between 60 and 68 degrees.

➤ Avoid TV and other blue light (computer screens) in your bedroom.

➤ Try to go to bed at the same time every night and get up at the same time every morning. You will create an internal sleep clock for yourself.

➤ Create a pre-sleep routine that does NOT include your phone or TV. Try reading a book, sipping a cup of tea, or meditating.

Take Action: If you feel your sleep quality is perfect, then (a) you are lucky(!), and (b) you can skip this action item. But, if not, choose at least one thing, if not more, from this list and focus on it this week. Continue to add more sleep tips to your daily routine until the quality of your sleep is where it should be. Feeling stuck? Sleep, or lack thereof, still leaving you fatigued (and really hungry) throughout the day? Well, remember for any of the topics discussed in this book, talking to your healthcare professionals makes good sense. Their suggestions might be just what you need.

Water

Dieting and sleeping aren't the only activities that can mess with your biology. Water ranks right up there as something worth paying attention to when trying to finally master weight management. Water is probably the second-best thing we can put into our bodies (after oxygen, of course!), yet a lot of people don't realize how truly valuable it can be—especially when they are trying to lose weight.

The term "water weight" gets tossed around a lot and can cause people to start drinking less water for fear of gaining back this dreaded water weight! The fact is that the exact opposite occurs when you drink water regularly. Here are some of the amazing impacts water can have on your weight management efforts:

> **Dehydration:** It is true that initial weight loss is often due to a loss of water. All the more reason you need to drink water, because when you lose all that "water weight," you become dehydrated. That water needs to be replaced for your body to function effectively and to avoid fatigue. Even mild dehydration can stop your weight-loss efforts dead in their tracks. When your body is properly hydrated and all your systems are functioning accordingly, you are most likely to lose weight efficiently.

> **Authentic appetite:** In general, the initial feelings of thirst and hunger are indistinguishable. You might be misinterpreting thirst as hunger and grabbing a snack when what you truly need is a glass of water. Drinking

water regularly helps avoid this problem by preventing thirst from sneaking up on you. Drinking water throughout the day and before meals ensures that you are not eating food out of thirst rather than true, physiological hunger. But, and this is an important but, you shouldn't use drinking water to temporarily "drown" your hunger and make it easier to stick to a diet. That's called water loading, and it's all about restricting your calories rather than learning to eat in response to your natural (rather than diet-driven) appetite.

> **Metabolism:** As mentioned above, dehydration slows your body's systems, causing them to work less effectively. One of the functions that is slowed with dehydration is the body's fat-burning system. However, when your body is well-hydrated and functioning appropriately, your metabolic rate will increase, helping you burn more calories and feel more energized. In fact, when your body is fully hydrated, your calorie burn rate can increase by as much as 30 percent!

> **Digestion and Toxin Removal:** Eating more fiber is often recommended for general health and digestive reasons; in fact, it is usually a big part of any weight-loss plan. However, if your body is not adequately hydrated you can lose all the beneficial effects of fiber in exchange for constipation! That's not much of a bargain! In addition, if you are burning calories, that process creates toxins in your body, and water is vital to help flush those toxins out.

> **Kidney Function:** Adequate water intake is essential for healthy kidney function. Without adequate hydration, your kidneys can flounder and that might put more stress on the liver. You might be wondering what this has to do with weight loss . . . well, a major function of the liver is

to help burn fat. So, if the liver is "distracted" by kidneys that aren't working effectively, fat burning ends up taking a backseat.

> **Water Retention:** Some people avoid water intake to prevent bloating and water retention. The problem with that is that water intake doesn't CAUSE water retention; it CURES it! When you drink water, the body realizes that it is now properly hydrated and sends the signal to let go of any water it was previously retaining. In other words, once it's hydrated, it no longer needs to retain water, and the bloat goes away!

Given the incredible benefits that drinking water can have on managing your weight without resorting to diets, it makes sense to brainstorm ways of increasing your water intake. Here are some of my favorite suggestions for making sure that your body is getting the water it needs:

> Drink a big glass of water 10 to 15 minutes before eating. This will help make sure you are eating out of hunger and not because you're dehydrated.

> Go to the water fountain every hour that you are at work.

> Replace sugary or artificially sweetened beverages with water. It will cut hundreds of calories from your day and/ or decrease the intake of chemicals that in some cases might interfere with weight loss.

> Drink a large glass of water when you first wake up in the morning. It will impact your eating and cravings for the rest of the day by ensuring that thirst isn't masquerading as hunger.

> Create hourly water goals. You can keep track of these goals by marking a refillable water bottle that you keep close by. It will be obvious that you haven't had enough to

drink when the level of water in the bottle isn't dropping as fast as it should be.

➢ If you don't like downing a whole glass of water at a single time, keep a water bottle with you all day and sip from it again and again and again!

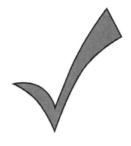

Take Action: If you haven't been drinking enough water on a regular basis, choose something from this list, or create your own, but commit to increasing your water intake this week. (Just make sure you don't increase it too much! Your healthcare professionals can provide you general guidelines for your recommended daily intake.) You might have to try several different techniques until you find the one(s) that click. But that's okay, this program is a work in progress and doesn't require that you "get it right" from the start. As your intake of water starts to catch up with your body's needs, not only will weight management get easier, but you'll likely feel more energetic and balanced.

Chronic Stress

Ah, yes, chronic stress. The state that far too many of us know far too much about. Sources of chronic stress are so wide and so varied, that you can take your pick of a seemingly infinite number of stressors: your recent job change, the manager at work who doesn't know the difference between constructive feedback and bullying, your pending move from apartment A to apartment B, the holidays, the construction on your street, the financial "crisis" that never seems to be out of the headlines . . . well, you get the idea. Knowing full well that stress is a reality of life, our bodies developed some nifty ways of managing.

Enter cortisol and other stress hormones, which in small doses for small amounts of time can help us to run faster, be stronger, and finally outsmart that wily saber-toothed tiger that's chasing us across the plains. But, wait a minute, nowadays we're not talking about short bursts of energy to get ourselves out of life-threatening situations. We're talking about hour after hour after hour of stress that sometimes doesn't let up for days, week, or even years! Now cortisol, a welcome guest for short periods of time, starts to overstay its welcome. And along with that comes an increase in appetite, weight gain that selectively goes to your belly (hello, visceral obesity), high blood sugar, and a slowed metabolism. Yikes! If there were ever reasons to address your stress as part of managing your weight—well, there they are.

Getting Biology on Your Side

Don't despair if you can't fix everything in your (biological) life that is making your appetite for French fries bigger than it's ever been. Babies will wake you at night, you might have chosen a profession that requires rotating shifts, inevitably you'll forget your water bottle in the car, and the economy isn't going to be all better anytime soon. The beauty of this program is that it doesn't require perfection, it doesn't require a "stress free" life to work. So, if less sleep than you need is going to be your reality for the foreseeable future, then try another skill. Maybe it's challenging the thought that "The only way I'm going to survive this shift is if I get something really sweet from the vending machine."

Maybe it's giving up an hour of screen time to take a nap. If it's the chronic stress of going to school while holding down a job (or two) that you're facing, then accept that your biology might be contributing to your weight problem and commit to being kind to yourself no matter what the scale says. At least that way you aren't adding guilt and shame to the mix. If you panicked and went back to dieting, accept that old habits die hard and nudge yourself back to the healthy eating (and healthy hormones) that this program brings.

But sometimes there are things we can do, even though they have escaped our attention up until now. In the hustle and bustle of daily life, we might have "normalized" things that really can change. Use the following worksheet to identify ways you can make biology your weight-management friend rather than your weight-management foe. If your sleep is just the way it should be, you can move on to chronic stress. If you don't have any of that . . . wait, who am I kidding? We all have chronic stress, so you're not getting out of that one. For that category, think of anything, big to small, that you can do to improve the things in life that make the daily grind so, well, grinding. And, as for returning to the dieting that helped trigger the yoyo in the first place, remind yourself that "doing the same thing over and over again and expecting a different result" doesn't make a lot of sense. I've given you some examples in the worksheet but make sure to customize it to your life.

BIOLOGICAL STRESSOR	POSSIBLE SOLUTIONS
Sleep: Not getting enough sleep – soooo tired in the morning.	1. No screen for at least two hours before bed (You'll survive, I promise!) 2. Make sure your room is very dark. Light from outside, from the digital alarm clock, and from the cell phone on your bedside table can keep your brain from settling down.
Chronic stress: Can't stop worrying – ever – about work.	1. Make yourself a worry book. Put down your thoughts in the book (instead of letting them go around and around your head). 2. Get support from a friend – brainstorm ways to make work better. 3. Ask yourself, "Will this job ever stop interfering with my health." If not, maybe you should start making an exit plan.
Dieting: Starting to diet "just a little" because summer is just around the corner.	1. Remind yourself that you've done this every summer for the last 15 years. And guess what, no matter how much you lost, you always gain backed 5 pounds more. 2. Ask yourself "Would I knowingly take a pill that would make my appetite feel out of control". If the answer is no, then why go back to the dieting that has done just that?
Hydration: Forgetting to drink water for most of the day.	1. Pair drinking water with routines you have throughout the day e.g. drink a glass of water when you brush your teeth; drink a glass of water after you walk the dog; drink a glass of water before each meal.

Take Action: Okay, now it's your turn. Remember that biological stressors don't only include dieting, hydration, sleep, and chronic stress. Pain, certain medical conditions (for example, low thyroid function), premenstrual syndrome (PMS), and time of the year (February blues, anyone?) are just some of the other biological factors that can contribute to an appetite gone wild. Take some time to think about your own situation and then brainstorm possible solutions, making sure that you keep your healthcare professionals informed of what you plan on doing. They might have their own solutions to suggest.

BIOLOGICAL STRESSOR	POSSIBLE SOLUTIONS

Case Study: Biology in Action

Sarah had been working shifts as a nurse for years. In her twenties, she could swing it without much of a problem. But now, in her late thirties, Sarah was finding her wonky sleep patterns hard to manage. When she was at work and needed to be alert and on her game, Sarah would use caffeine (sometimes coffee, sometimes soda, sometimes both) to make it through the night. Never a bottle of water, because it just didn't have any "buzz" to offer.

Even so, caffeine loading wasn't enough for Sarah most of the time. That's why she'd find herself using food to get through the night. And the food she was using wasn't leafy green salads and avocado toast. It was all about cookies, chips, and anything else she could find in the vending machine. But it wasn't about a few cookies or a single bag of chips, it was about a steady stream of food (if we can call it that)! Sarah felt like she was a bottomless pit. By the end of the shift, she was tired yet wired (thanks, caffeine), and felt so bloated and heavy (although, even then, she would have still made room for another serving of . . . well, anything. That's how crazy her appetite felt).

The irony of being a healthcare professional who wasn't taking care of her own health hadn't escaped Sarah. For years now, Sarah had given up on living any other way. She figured she was just one of those people who didn't have the drive or determination to stick to her diet plan. (Sarah seemed to forget that she had both drive and determination to spare in other parts of her life. She had excelled in nursing school, she was a great mom who made time for her kids at every opportunity, and she was an outstanding advocate for her patients.)

After putting some focus on changing, Sarah began to consider the possibility that her "lack of willpower" was really "lack of sleep," and she began to view herself differently. Maybe she wasn't a write-off when it came to her own health. Maybe there was a way out of this pattern of eating her way through her shifts. Sarah began by logging her daily hours of sleep—a whopping total of four to five hours per night. Not nearly enough. Some days that was the best Sarah could do when balancing her other priorities.

Realizing that investing in her own health would be in her family's best interest (so, no, it wasn't selfish), Sarah starting to protect time for napping or going to bed sooner, rather than later. It wasn't a miracle cure, but after a few weeks with an hour or two of extra sleep a day, Sarah noticed that her appetite wasn't so out of control at work. She also gave some thought to her snacks— not because she was restricting food, but because she didn't want to add all-over-the-place blood sugar to her list of "biological factors" that were making it even harder to lose weight.

Yes, sometimes she snacked on Oreos, but she also took her favorite healthy treats to work. (And favorite is an important point—she didn't try to replace "junk" food with healthy food that she could barely stand. Sarah went out of the way to make sure she would enjoy her snacks. What that meant was fresh mango, guacamole, and brazil nuts. What it didn't mean was a bag of tasteless and on-the-dry side mini carrots).

Better sleep, better nutrition, and easing up on herself made a difference to Sarah. ("Oh, there's an urge to eat a lot of food right now. I must be tired" replaced "Oh, I'm so pathetic—I want to eat everything again!") And, slowly but surely, the weight that hadn't done anything but go up throughout the years, began to plateau and, eventually, move in the opposite direction. This wasn't all thanks to biology, as Sarah used the whole Shatter the Yoyo program. Still, improving her sleep clearly helped Sarah manage her weight successfully for the first time in years.

Bottom Line

Biology can make your appetite seem out of control. If that's what's going on, then forget lecturing yourself about willpower. (In fact, even if that's not what's going on, forget about lecturing yourself about willpower. If that worked, there wouldn't be a bad habit in sight!)

Instead, do your best to get enough sleep, drink enough water, reduce your chronic stress, and to stay far, far away from the dieting that has helped keep the yoyo alive and well. Addressing these parts of your life won't solve the thinking or feeling parts of the yoyo pattern (that's what the rest of the program is for), but it will stop making weight management that much harder.

Change Your Focus

CHAPTER 6

Are You Focusing on the Right Things?

"When you stop chasing the wrong things, you give the right things a chance to catch you."

—LOLLY DASKAL

The first step in this program is to identify your current focus and, if need be, change it to something that will help you achieve your weight-management goals. If you're like most dieters, chances are that your dominant thoughts about your weight have been the same for a long time. These thoughts are along the lines of, "I need to go back on a diet" or "The only way for me to lose weight is to be on a diet." Often these thoughts have been further entrenched by friends or family members who have bought into the you-have-to-diet-if-you-ever-expect-to-lose-weight school of thought.

For me, it was always "The only way to lose weight is to count calories." Once upon a time that was my mantra, and it was the only thing I focused on, meal after meal, day after day. I didn't know there was any other way to manage my weight, so I didn't even realize there was a reason to change my focus. Once I realized that dieting was never going to work for me, I changed my focus and, just like that, it felt like a lot more changed in my life. I no longer felt dependent and helpless. In fact, it was quite the opposite. I felt powerful, in control, and like I could do anything! And it all started with a shift in focus—a change of perspective on what I needed to do to solve my weight problem for good.

Changing your focus is a bit like putting on polarized sunglasses. They might not change your vision, but they allow you to see things in a different way. And when you see things differently, your associated thoughts and feelings tend to change also. There is a common expression in yoga: "Where your eyes go, your body with follow." This is what is happening when you change your focus—you are moving yourself in a different direction.

The time has come to focus on your change in perspective. You might be reading this because you want to lose weight or simply manage your weight—but, in this program those goals are meant to be maintained for the long-term. This is different from all your previous diets, which were about focusing on losing weight right here, right now. That's perspective shift number one.

In addition, this program is about focusing on change that isn't extreme. Instead it should be realistic, manageable, and sustainable. That means none of that "lose weight quick" nonsense. This program is about permanently losing weight in a healthy and sustainable way. And that means SLOWLY—perspective shift number two. Not quite like all the programs that promise quick and extreme weight loss, wouldn't you agree?

Maybe you've seen the report about *The Biggest Loser* TV show and how several of the winners regained all the weight (and then some) that they lost. The report talked about resting metabolic rate and the risks of eating so little that your metabolism comes to a grinding halt. A diet program that promises that you will lose lots of weight, and you'll lose it fast, is a great business model. The cycle of weight loss and weight gain mostly guarantees repeat customers.

The Shatter the Yoyo program is different. For one, I'm not looking for repeat customers. I'm looking to help you overcome eating and weight problems once and for all. This program is also not about extreme, quick weight loss. Instead, it takes the slow but sure approach to weight management.

Three Steps to Changing Your Focus

Now let's get into the meat of changing your focus. As we delve deeper into this program, keep in mind that changing your focus is a three-step process:

- ➢ Step 1. Explore
- ➢ Step 2. Expand
- ➢ Step 3. Exchange

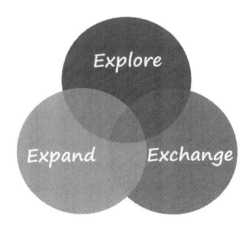

Exploring Your Diet Mentality

We start this step by looking at your goals. When you really explore what dieting is about for you and what you are hoping to achieve by losing weight, you can connect with your authentic motivation. This then allows you to focus on it in a healthy way.

Next, this program helps you identify the beliefs and behaviors that are from your previous diets. For example, the belief that you must restrict yourself from eating certain foods (usually some of your favorite treats) if you ever want to lose weight is a common holdover from years of dieting.

Having identified these "diet" thoughts and behaviors, you will gain the skills needed to leave them behind and make room for thoughts and behaviors that support lasting weight loss. Last, in this step, we look at the "diet language" that has become completely automatic after going through the cycle of weight loss and weight gain so many times. You will work on changing this language to support your determination to lose weight once and for all without falling back on old, extreme, and short-term dieting techniques.

To illustrate why this step is so important to the success of this program, let me give you an example of how diets can linger. I worked with a client, Diane, who had done the Weight Watchers program approximately 16 times. I say "approximately," because Diane had done it so many times that, honestly, she had lost track of the number of attempts. When it came to food, eating, and weight, it was all she knew. That program created her focus and defined her perspective. Diane only saw food in terms of "points." And she knew exactly how many points EVERYTHING was and was ALWAYS counting them—even though she wasn't even aware she was always doing it.

Yep, point counting had been automatic for Diane, even though people who are naturally thin, who have never had to worry about their weight, never, never count points. They would probably think I was crazy if I tried to explain to them why they needed to use points to decide what and what not to eat. If Diane wanted to achieve lasting weight loss, she needed to model herself after those who are naturally thin, not those who need a diet to "control" their urge to eat.

It was a huge struggle for Diane to change her perspective and shift away from asking, "How many points?" are in this food and that food. These thoughts were automatic for her, so it was an uphill battle to change her thinking in this regard. She worked really hard at it and, once her perspective truly started to change, other changes started to roll into Diane's life. And not only changes to her weight. Sure, she lost weight and kept it off, and that was an amazing accomplishment for Diane.

But things also changed in other aspects of Diane's life. She felt more relaxed at home with her kids, she felt more driven and motivated at work, and she felt more appreciative of her time with her husband. It was almost as if letting go of that old focus allowed Diane to open up and grow in many other ways. By freeing up some of her "head space" for other thoughts and feelings, giving up dieting allowed Diane to develop a deep appreciation for aspects of life that previously had been lost in a haze of sadness and frustration about her weight. Diane truly felt like she was getting her life back.

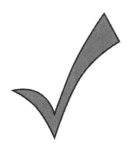

Take Action: So, now it's your turn—where has your focus been during the years that you have been yoyo dieting? What diet perspectives are now with you wherever you go? Take some time to think about the food and weight-related thoughts and behaviors you developed since you started dieting. Identify them on the worksheet and refer to them later when you are working on changing the unhealthy focus and perspectives caused by diet after diet.

Old Diet Thoughts

_____
_____
_____
_____
_____
_____
_____
_____
_____
_____
_____
_____
_____
_____
_____

Old Diet Behaviors

_____
_____
_____
_____
_____
_____
_____
_____
_____
_____
_____
_____
_____
_____
_____

CHAPTER 7

Focusing on the Goals of Your Goals

"There's only one corner of the universe you can be certain of improving, and that's your own self."

—ALDOUS HUXLEY

When I first started to focus on dieting, if anyone had asked me what my goal was, I would have said, "to lose weight." I mean, wasn't that kind of obvious? Why else would anyone go on a diet? I was convinced that what I wanted to get from all my efforts was weight loss. I never bothered to dig any deeper or look at my real motivation. And, why would I? Isn't wanting weight loss enough?

Well, it turns out it wasn't enough for me, and that's one of the reasons I was never able to stick with any "eating program" for the long term. It was also one of the reasons I wasn't able to maintain my weight loss—because it truly didn't mean enough to me. It was a generic goal, shared by millions (billions?), but there was no depth or personalization to it. For me, wanting to lose weight wasn't something I connected to emotionally on a deep level. Sure, there was some emotion involved, because I was unhappy with my weight and excited about the prospect of losing weight quickly. But these emotions didn't run deep enough for me. Losing weight had as much depth as saying, "I want to go pick up my dry cleaning."

At the time, had you followed up my explanation that I wanted to lose weight with the question, "Why?" I think I would have been dumbfounded. I wouldn't have had an answer. Or I might have come back with something snarky like, "What do you mean why? Doesn't everybody? Isn't it a normal goal?" And while that might be true, a deep and personal "why" is what I was missing.

The "why" that was important was the why that would explain the true meanings and emotions behind my determination to lose weight. When I finally did start examining my own personal "whys" instead of parroting the typical answer, I quickly realized that it wasn't true that I simply wanted to lose weight. It was really that I wanted to feel independent and in control of my body. I wanted to feel like I didn't need someone else or some program to tell me what I should be eating at every meal and every snack. And I really didn't want to feel like I was going to have to go back to dieting again and again. That was a kind of dependence I knew I didn't want for the rest of my life. I wanted to feel strong and in control in my relationship with food. I wanted to be the one who was calling the shots, not a piece of paper with rules about eating and exercise. That realization was everything for me. It represents what I now call "The Goals of Your Goals™."

I am hopeful that this realization will be equally powerful for you. I suspect that most of you are just like I was; focused on the goal of losing weight, without being aware of your deeper, personal reasons for wanting to weigh less. And without knowing the deeper reasons, your weight-loss goal just won't have the same power or drive behind it.

This is the first focus change you will be making as part of the Shatter the Yoyo program. You will be looking at losing weight as a starting point, not as an endpoint. Most people reading this book have the same goals—either to lose weight or to maintain weight loss and not have to diet anymore. So, those particular goals are now the **what**—as in "What do I want to accomplish by doing this program?"

The what is important and can be a useful initial driver. But the what is not everything, and it is definitely not the core power that will help you make healthy, sustainable changes to your eating and weight. Relying only on the what likely helps to explain why you haven't had success achieving and/or maintaining weight loss in the past.

This program is much more about **why** weight loss is important to you—the changes to your life you believe will come along with losing weight. In my opinion, the why is the real motivation and fuel you will need to finally achieve your weight-management goals.

So, what are the whys? Well, they are the reasons behind your weight-loss/weight-management goals. In other words, they are the benefits you expect from finally being able to manage your weight to your own satisfaction. The whys are also the impediments that you lose as a result of reaching your goals. Taken together, you could say that the whys are the way your life changes for the better because of losing weight and keeping it off.

You want to lose weight? You want to be done with dieting? And, you want to stop yoyo dieting? Of course, you do! Those are great goals . . . but why? Why do you want to do all those things? Most of us have those goals in common, but the whys can be different. The whys can cover a variety of different areas: health, confidence, body image, self-esteem, self-image, work, relationships, playtime, and family, to name just a few.

There is no wrong why. If your why is because you want to feel confident in a swimsuit, well, that is no more or less important than someone else's why of wanting to control their diabetes. The best why for you reflects what drives you! It doesn't reflect what drives your parents, siblings, friends, colleagues, or strangers at the gym. Below are some of the personalized reasons for weight loss that you might discover when you take the time to identify the goals of your weight-loss goal (aka The Goals of Your Goals).

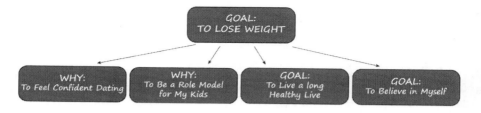

For most of us, The Goals of Your Goals is a list, not a single item. Because of that, this list might cover several areas. You might want to lose weight to feel more confident in your career and your sex life, to feel more comfortable in your clothes, and to not feel physically held back. You might want to lose weight to ensure that you live a long and healthy life, to ensure you are able to play in the park with your children, to be able to smile when you look in the mirror, and to be more confident and engaged socially. Let me say it again: There are no wrong whys!

Here are some examples of The Goals of Your Goals from actual clients:

- I will be able to be more active.
- I will have more confidence.
- I will teach my children how to be healthy.
- I will be the person I know I can be.

- I will be proud of myself.
- I will dress to show off instead of cover-up.
- I will reduce my risk for diabetes and other illnesses.
- I will have more energy.
- My life will be more balanced.
- I will be more social.
- I won't always be worried about food.
- I will be more comfortable in my own skin.
- I will be able to borrow my friend's clothes.
- I'll enjoy physical intimacy more.
- I will be more comfortable eating in front of people.
- I won't live my life in fear of being judged.
- I will be able to cross my legs.
- I will stop calling myself names.
- I will be comfortable in a bathing suit.
- I will enjoy shopping.
- I will finally have the confidence to ask for that promotion.
- I will stop avoiding dating.
- I will be able to speak up in my marriage.

Again, as you can see from these examples, there are no wrong answers; it is simply what drives you. And I want to make sure that you are crystal clear on why you are so driven to lose weight, so you can use it as a powerful source of true motivation. That kind of motivation comes in handy when the work required to give up dieting feels a lot harder than you expected. That happens, it's normal, but being motivated by your own personal collection of whys makes getting through the difficult times, that much easier.

It might have occurred to you that these goals could also be reasons for dieting—we all know that diets can result in short-term weight loss. That they "work" is what makes diets such a big industry. So, sure, a diet can make you feel more comfortable in a bathing suit or help you feel more social. The problem is that these benefits don't last for most people. So, keep in mind that the list of your own personal whys reflects what you want to achieve for the long term. This list should not be about what you want to achieve for a two-week period in August (the two-week period right before you fall off the diet wagon and find yourself knee deep in potato chips)!

 **Take Action:** Here is your next action item. I want you to create your list of whys, The Goals of Your Goals list. Using the next page, sit down with your favorite pen, and start brainstorming about what is truly driving your desire to lose weight. You might have a few answers that have already come to mind while reading this chapter, and you might have a few others that quickly come up as you sit with it. There might be a lot more whys below the surface, so carve out some time for this exercise to make sure you aren't missing anything. Asking yourself some questions can sometimes help you uncover the true whys behind your weight loss efforts:

➤ Have you lost weight before?
➤ If so, how did you feel?
➤ How was your life, your perspective, your attitude different when you lost weight?
➤ How did you feel when you gained the weight back?
➤ What changed when you gained the weight back? Was it an activity? A relationship? A different self-perspective?

> ➤ What are you afraid of?
> ➤ What do you truly want?
> ➤ How is your weight holding you back?

Once you feel your list is complete, I want you to make a commitment to **read it every day**. Yes, I did say, "every day!" I want you to stay connected to these whys, The Goals of Your Goals and really engrain them in your brain. This way you will always remember why you are willing to put so much time and energy into completing this program and achieving your weight-management goals.

Put your list of whys in your smartphone, on your bathroom mirror, near your coffeemaker, or on your nightstand. Put the list wherever it needs to be so that you don't forget to review it daily. Make reading this list part of your daily routine until you've completed this book, settled into the program, and are making steady progress. Reviewing this list repeatedly is a way of staying connected to what really drives you. And this connection will keep you moving forward, even when you are feel discouraged and begin to contemplate another round of yoyo dieting.

The Goals of Your Goals

Goal #1 _____

_____

Goal #2 _____

_____

Goal #3 _____

_____

Goal #4 _____

_____

Goal #5 _____

_____

Goal #6 _____

_____

Goal #7 _____

_____

Goal #8 _____

_____

Goal #9 _____

_____

CHAPTER 8

From Restriction to Permission (Yes, Ice Cream Can Really Be a Regular Part of Your Life)

"He who controls others might be powerful, but he who has mastered himself is mightier still."

—LAO TZU

Here's something you should know about me—I love ice cream. I mean really love ice cream. I would list it as my absolute favorite thing to eat. As a child, I think it was rare for more than a day to pass without me having a heaping bowl of chocolate ice cream. And, often, it wasn't just a single serving. Instead I'd be sitting down to a ton of my favorite flavors! Of course, back then I didn't have any concern about weight gain or health, so eating a half gallon of ice cream every day wasn't really a problem, believe it or not.

Alternatively, when I first started to focus on weight loss and my "calorie counting is all that matters" philosophy, ice cream immediately fell on the naughty list. I basically decided that I could never have ice cream again. But, surprise, surprise, that's not actually how things turned out. I certainly didn't end up giving up ice cream once and for all. I mean, why I even expected to do that when I loved ice cream so much is beyond me.

So, can you guess what happened when I was exposed to ice cream again after imposing a "never eat ice cream" rule on myself? I went hog wild, that's what. Instead of stopping at a single bowl or cone, I just ate all of it! If I bought a pint, I ate a pint. If I bought a half gallon, I ate a half gallon. It was as if I had completely lost the ability to control my intake of ice cream.

How could it be that a full-grown adult was powerless over ice cream? Once I gave up dieting, I could answer that question quite easily. By making ice cream a forever "bad" food that was off-limits, I felt incredibly deprived and restricted. Naturally, when I finally did allow myself that indulgence, I went way overboard. It was as if I didn't know when I might ever get the chance to eat ice cream again, so I was going to enjoy every bit of it that I could. And boy, did I!

This is a really great example of how RESTRICTION = POWER™. When you restrict foods, or put them on your no-no list, you basically give them absolute power over you. They consume your thoughts, and ultimately set you up for binge-eating behavior. My eating a gallon of cream at a single sitting is evidence of just that!

You are probably familiar with this concept of off-limits foods. Most people, and most every dieter out there, have them. These are the foods that you are convinced you can't have in the house or even have anywhere around you without completely losing control and eating every bite. My guess is that your list of off-limits foods keeps growing! But the real problem with these foods is not how much we eat them. The problem is that by making them off-limits, you hand over a lot of power to these foods. At the same time, you are giving yourself a strong message that your self-control isn't enough to keep you "safe" around cookies, donuts, fried chicken, or whatever happens to be your "weakness."

I'm willing to guess that most of you would probably swear up and down that you have absolutely no control around your off-limits foods. Well, I'm here to argue otherwise. Whether you eat a slice of pizza or a whole pizza is always a choice that you have the power to make. But you make the choice a lot harder when you add restriction to the mix. Suddenly both your psychology (that is, wanting what you can't have) and your biology (that is, wanting to fight back against a "famine") point you in the direction of frantically eating the whole pizza, rather than just enough slices to leave you feeling satisfied rather than stuffed.

It becomes a vicious cycle. You think you have no control, so you restrict certain foods. This deprivation sets you up to binge on high-calorie, high-fat, high-sugar foods, which just confirms to you that you have no control. So, now you try even harder to restrict your intake of "fattening foods," and round and round you go. The list of restricted foods gets longer, and the binges get bigger. I know a lot of people who have lived that nightmare. It's crazy making! The thing is, it doesn't have to be that way.

The restriction/binge cycle can be broken. But it can't be broken by trying to come up with bigger and better ways to keep yourself from eating off-limits foods. It can only be broken by doing the exact opposite—letting yourself eat the ice cream that seems to call your name from the freezer or the buttery cinnamon rolls that you haven't "allowed" yourself to eat for the past 10 years. (Although that hasn't stopped you from bingeing on them!)

At first you are likely to go overboard. Welcome to "catch-up eating," something that occurs when you truly give yourself permission to eat and enjoy off-limits foods. You are so used to the foods being in limited supply, that your old habit of eating as much as you can of the ice cream before it is put back on the restricted list will take some time to change. But once you demonstrate to your mind and body that you are serious about never, ever again making any food off-limits, you won't have the drive to "get while the getting is good."

Then one day, to your utter surprise, you'll find yourself putting the pint of chocolate chip cookie dough ice cream back in the freezer after a single serving without giving it even a second thought. Eventually you might even discover that some of your off-limits foods aren't as exciting or even as tasty as you thought they were. I've had more than a few clients who for years binged on foods like hamburgers, French fries, and chips, only to discover that, meh, they weren't their favorite foods after all. By eliminating restrictions and rules about food, you will open the door to your authentic likes and loves, rather than being a "reactive" eater.

The fact is that there is no such thing as *bad* food. Ice cream certainly isn't on the list of the top ten healthy foods, but it's not a bad food either. Especially if you're just eating it out of true hunger and not because you're bored, tired, or rebelling against a diet. Ice cream only became a problem for me when I restricted it. Once I realized this, I knew something had to change. So, I made a plan—I was going to go to the ice cream shop once a week and treat myself. I looked forward to that ice cream shop all week, and I thoroughly enjoyed every bite, but I never binged or ate ice cream in an out-of-control way. I knew I got to have it every week and simply knowing that was enough to keep me content.

After a while of reintroducing ice cream into my life like this, I started keeping single-serving ice cream containers or bars in the house. My routine was to have them two or three times a week. Eventually I graduated to having pints of ice cream in the house. Now, it's okay. I know how much I need to feel satisfied rather than uncomfortably full. I know ice cream is not bad, and I know

I'm allowed to have it now and in the future. Allowing myself to have ice cream is not a time-limited offer. Ice cream might be a permanent part of my diet-free life, but it has no power and no control over me.

Now, let's say pizza is your top no-no food. I'm not suggesting that you fill your house with pizza and go crazy on a pizza-eating spree. But I am suggesting that you get rid of the off-limits foods list and start incorporating these foods back into your diet in a healthy way. Again, using pizza as the example, why not plan to start eating pizza twice a week? This will immediately remove the stigma you have associated with eating pizza. ("Oh, no, I've blown it again. I'm eating pizza! I can't believe how little control I have over it!")

It also means that you have removed the "restricted" label from pizza. By removing that label, you have also begun the process of removing the drive to eat all eight pieces the next time an opportunity to eat pizza comes up (because it came up so infrequently and you never knew when the next opportunity would be!) Formerly an off-limits food, pizza is now a food that is available to you and which you can have regularly, if you so choose.

By allowing it into your life, you are taking away the power that pizza used to have over your eating behavior. In addition, if you are familiar with aspects of mindful eating, the meals in which you incorporate your "no-no" foods will be a great opportunity to focus on mindfulness. This will help you to truly appreciate and savor all the aspects of eating and enjoying that food. If you are not familiar with mindful eating, it is something I discuss in-depth in my full online Shatter the Yoyo Program.

When looking at the concept of restriction, it's also important to point out how much more valuable it is for the psyche to focus on the positive instead of the negative. When it comes to dieting, there is a lot of emphasis on foods that are not allowed. Whether it is carbs, fats, sugar, or ice cream, you tell yourself that you can't have these foods, and the next thing you know they're all you can think about.

Dieting has brought with it a hyperfocus on "forbidden" foods. Wouldn't it feel so much better to focus on all the good foods out there? Think about the positives and all the delicious things you can eat that truly nourish your body? Personally, I'd much rather think about sweet potatoes, cashews, and strawberries, than focus on things I'm "not allowed" to eat!

Let me give you an example of how this applied to a former client of mine. When Allison first came to my office she was a 31-year-old yoga instructor who spent some evenings and weekends working for a catering business. Allison had been a model in her late teens and early twenties, which meant she had been focusing on her body and keeping her weight down for years.

If you asked any of Allison's yoga students about her, they would have probably told you that Allison was one of the healthiest people they knew. There, in my office, it was clear that Allison was in great shape and physically fit. Allison was also health conscious when it came to food and used to take all sorts of delicious homemade protein bars to yoga class for her students.

Allison was upbeat, engaging, and full of what you could call a "positive attitude." But what Allison's students didn't realize was that she has been yoyo dieting ever since she went on her first diet at age 16. For years, Allison had been trying this diet and that diet, and they were all successful for the short-term.

The problem for Allison was the restriction. For example, prior to starting my program, Allison's last diet had been low-carb. That meant that she was eating absolutely no grains and limited fruits and even some vegetables. Allison did really well with this diet for about three weeks until her next catering gig. As Allison was cleaning up at the end of the night, she came face-to-face with a bag of rolls, and the next thing she knew she was working her way through all 40 of them. I'm sure you know that is excessive.

Such is the power of restriction to make people do things they would never have considered doing before they started dieting. Feeling frantic and not wanting to be "caught," Alison took the bag into the bathroom and ate the entire thing in about five minutes. And then there she was, feeling sick, ashamed, and scared of how little self-control she seemed to have. Before going on this low-carb diet, Allison had never had a problem with overeating bread. It wasn't until she introduced that particular restriction that bread, pasta, crackers, and potatoes gained an incredible amount of power over her eating behavior.

Something similar happened to Allison on a previous diet that required her to completely eliminate fruit from her eating plan. A couple of weeks into this diet, Allison found herself bingeing on a massive amount of fruit. As a result, Allison had to spend about twelve hours in the bathroom because her stomach was so upset! Again, clearly the restriction was the problem. When I met Allison, she was on the low carb diet and was bingeing regularly on carbs. Still, Allison didn't want to stop the low carb diet because she was scared her weight would skyrocket. (Of course, it was restricting the carbs in the first place that left Allison at risk of weight gain from bingeing. But even knowing that intellectually, emotionally Allison's fear of weight gain wouldn't let her ditch the low carb diet entirely).

So, here's what we did: Each day we had Allison eat a bread product (a roll, pastry, croissant, toast, whatever), and then maintain her low carb diet for the rest of the day. It worked perfectly! In the beginning, Allison found that all she could think about was what bread product she was going to have for breakfast the next day. But after about a week or so, her thoughts about breakfast stopped being so compulsive. It just became a typical part of her daily routine. There was no more restriction, so there was no more power. To date, Allison has not binged in seven months.

 **Take Action:** If you are going to follow in Allison's footsteps, the first thing you will need to do is to identify all your off-limits foods. You might have one, you might have one hundred. Doesn't matter. Think about every food that you consider to be "no-no" or off-limits. Once you think this list is complete, go through it and pick one food to start with. Next, create a plan to regularly incorporate this food into your diet. It can be pizza once a week, a piece of chocolate every night, or avocado with breakfast a few times a week.

It's up to you but it must be *allowed*, and allowed without guilt, second-guessing or panic. That's important, because it's only when you are truly comfortable eating a food that it loses its power to trigger a binge. (And on that point, let's be clear. It isn't really the food that has the power. It's the biological and psychological drive that is triggered by restriction that has the power. It just feels like it's the food that is calling the shots, even though it's really *restricting* the food that unravels your ability to eat moderately. But identifying food as having the power is a convenient shorthand for this process).

My Off-Limits Foods

1) _____

2) _____

3) _____

4) _____

5) _____

6) _____

7) _____

8) _____

9) _____

10) _____

11) _____

12) _____

13) _____

14) _____

15) _____

The food I will start with is: _____

_____

My incorporation plan is: _____

_____

CHAPTER 9

Saying Goodbye to Our Diet Language

"I am beginning to measure myself in strength, not pounds. Sometimes in smiles."

—LAURIE HALSE ANDERSON

Earlier I mentioned my previous mindset of being solely focused on counting calories. Because of this hyperfocus on calories, I ignored the other aspects of virtually everything else I ate. Fat, protein, carbohydrate, sodium, flavor, how much I even liked the food, the individual ingredients—these were all nonissues for me. The only thing I focused on was calorie count. I had a finite diet language and my most used word was calorie. Other words that came up often in my vocabulary included "diet" (as in "I'm on a diet," or "I can't eat that on this diet.") and "cheat" (as in "I'm not supposed to be eating this, so I'm cheating"). Because of this diet language, my focus was on dieting and dieting alone. This was a type of thinking that I would eventually need to change to truly succeed at creating a diet-free life.

I spoke earlier about the value of changing your focus. One of the primary reasons for changing your focus is to look at this program as a long-term lifestyle change and not something you are doing temporarily. Shattering the Yoyo is not about losing 10 pounds quickly for an upcoming wedding. It is not about banning all carbohydrates for a month or doing a weeklong cleanse. And it is definitely not about eating only vegetables until beach season. Shattering the Yoyo is about embracing a real and sustainable lifestyle change that doesn't require extreme effort, rules, or regulations.

Unlike this program, the main problem with the diet mentality and the diet language I mentioned above, is that they are all temporary. The big question is not whether you can lose weight or not (yep, you sure can, as you have probably demonstrated again and again). The big question is, "What happens when you stop dieting?" Almost always, the weight comes right back (but you already knew that, didn't you?) And if you've been extremely restrictive with calories or food omissions, the weight comes back quickly and you might even end up heavier than when you started.

This is exactly how certain diet programs thrive. They hook people by helping them lose weight, but only for the short term. The "successful" dieter then either voluntarily or involuntarily stops dieting and gains all the weight back. And what do you think happens next? Often the person goes right back to the commercial diet program that most recently helped him or her lose weight. Maybe that helps explain why some popular commercial diet programs have more than 84 percent repeat customers! Great business model, right?

I'm guessing you don't want to be one of those 84 percent. I'm also guessing you don't want to have to go back on a diet again and constantly battle back and forth with your weight. If I'm right, you need to ditch that diet outlook and understand that you are making lifelong changes, not just changes that last until you've finished this program. I haven't designed this program for short-term success. Instead it helps you build a lifestyle that's not *extreme, rigid,* or *restrictive*. You'll learn a way of eating and managing your weight that is balanced, flexible, and healthy.

If you are going to successfully ditch that temporary diet outlook, then you also need to ditch your diet language. This is the language that keeps you focused on all the aspects of a diet that are temporary and don't represent a new lifestyle. Your diet language might include the word calories, as mine did. But it might also include related words and phrases, such as points, fat, good versus bad foods, carbs, cheats, macros, allowed, on a health kick, and off the diet. Can you think of others? For many dieters, these words are a way of life. But they are also words that keep you diet-focused, and ultimately stuck in the short-term, temporary-diet mentality.

You will definitely need to get rid of this diet language! The goal will be for you replace it with nondiet words, such as healthy, fresh, *real food*, hunger, and satiation. For me, my replacement language for calorie was real food. Instead of focusing on how many calories something had, I simply focused on whether it was a whole food and/or made of natural ingredients, instead of chemicals and fillers. For you, it might be about replacing the word *points* with the term *health value* or replacing *carb counting* with focusing on *getting more* fiber. Whatever it is, you need to stop using your old diet language, as it is part of what keeps you stuck on the yoyo diet seesaw.

Below are some examples of common diet language terms and their most frequent thought associations. I've also included suggested replacement (or new) language.

DIET LANGUAGE	ASSOCIATION	NEW LANGUAGE
Calories	Tracking/Monitoring	Healthy
Fat	Restriction	Nutritious
Carbs	Off Limits	Fiber
Cheat	Not Allowed	80/20 mentality

Now, how do you implement this diet language change? One of my favorite techniques for ditching the diet language is the swear-jar technique. I'm sure you are familiar with this—the jar that sits on the counter and anyone in the house who swears must throw a dollar in it. You can do the SAME thing for diet language! If you have other people in your household, include them to make you accountable. Have them point out anytime you use your old diet language.

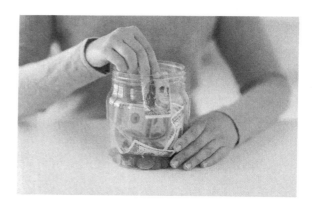

If you live alone, just make a point to pay attention to your language around food and hold yourself accountable to putting money in the jar. It might take a while, but you will start to catch yourself before you say things, and you will start using new language that supports your diet-free life. Use the money collected for some self-care—maybe a massage, a personal training session, a health-foods shopping spree—something good and healthy!

Generally, if you use diet language a lot, you are at greater risk of have a rigid, black-and-white way of thinking. This often manifests in the need to do everything right, with 100 percent effort. Nothing less than perfection will do. This is a type of all-or-nothing thinking (which we will talk about later), and, unfortunately, it sets you up for failure.

The reality is that no one can function at 100 percent all the time. It simply is not possible. You need wiggle room, you need space, and you need flexibility. You also need the option to deviate from your plan without stepping into the "I've blown it" trap and giving up on this program. Functioning at 100 percent capacity all the time is not an option—even though you might have been living your life as if it is a real possibility.

I am a firm believer in the 80/20 mentality. Put simply, the 80/20 approach to life means trying to stick with your plans 80 percent of the time. Sure, go ahead and shoot for 100 percent compliance, but remember it's extremely important to be okay with only hitting your target 80 percent of the time. The other 20 percent of the time, you can relax and let up a bit. And in keeping with this program's anti-perfectionism approach to weight management, the 80/20 split doesn't need to be exact.

If you feel it is important for you to not eat dinner out, and you eat dinner out one time a week, no big deal, that's close enough to 20 percent. If you feel you want to eat breakfast every day within an hour of waking, and every now and then you forget, or you are too rushed, no big deal—there's your 20 percent again. If you want to exercise every day and you find yourself missing a day, don't panic. Including 20 percent wiggle room in your life is an important part of this program. The idea is that you are striving to meet your goals or ideals *most* of the time, instead of all the time—there is a big difference between those words!

With rigid, 100-percent thinking, any deviation from your plans is a failure. And given that life never goes completely as planned, "failure" will happen again and again. Repeatedly feeling as if you have failed is an effective way to make you want to stop trying, give up, and fall back into old thinking patterns and behaviors. When you feel like you have failed (again!) or, even worse, feel like you, yourself, are a failure, it makes it a lot more likely that you will give up on your goals and plans. It's why so many people say, "I blew it—I'll just start again on Monday," when they have eaten an off-limits food or had an extra serving at dinner. This "what-the-hell-effect" drives many destructive overeating episodes. With the 80/20 mentality, there is no blowing it. There is just a steady attempt to reach your goals at least 80 percent of the time.

Of course, it is hard to include the 80/20 approach in your typical "lose weight fast" diet. Because the goal is to lose a substantial amount of weight and to lose it quickly, there is no wiggle room. The 20 percent wiggle room will wreak havoc on an extreme diet. For example, if you have a diet goal of losing 10 pounds in three weeks, sticking to the diet 100 percent of the time becomes necessary, because the goal is so extreme.

Breaking away from that type of rigidity and embracing this program with its healthy and sustainable eating and weight-management goals allows the 80/20 rule to fit in nicely! Moving away from black-and-white thinking toward an 80/20 mentality is a necessary change, if you want to shatter the yoyo once and for all!

Take Action: Now, here is your next assignment: Identify your own personal diet language and come up with replacement words. Make sure the 80/20 mentality is a part of your new health language. Then institute your own personal "swear jar" and come up with a reward for the money!

MY DIET LANGUAGE	MY REPLACEMENT LANGUAGE

Change Your Thoughts

CHAPTER 10

Understanding Automatic Thoughts

"You have power over your mind—not outside events. Realize this, and you will find strength."

—MARCUS AURELIUS

By this point in the program, you will have changed your focus and are looking at things through a new lens. You have developed a healthier perspective on weight management and food. The next step is to take a long, hard look at your thinking. Why is this important? Because most people have a tendency to think that when a situation changes, or becomes difficult or stressful, that the situation is to blame for the unhappiness, anger, or emotional discomfort that results. But psychological science tells us otherwise. It is the way a person **thinks** about a situation that invokes his or her emotional response, not the situation itself. This is known as the A-B-C model in cognitive psychology, and we're going to take a closer look at this concept right now.

Let's think of A as an *activating* event. In other words, it is something that happens to you. B is your *belief* or thoughts about what happened to you. Finally, C are the *consequences* or outcomes. The most commonly held idea is expressed like this:

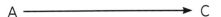

A ⟶ C

Simply, put, something happens (A, an activating event), and then there is an outcome of that event (C, the consequences). For example, you eat three pieces of apple pie instead of one (event A), and as a result you feel miserable and ashamed (consequence C).

The ABC model looks a little bit different:

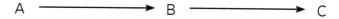

A ⟶ B ⟶ C

What this model suggests is that something happens (A, an activating event) and there are thoughts about this event (B, a belief), and it is those thoughts that truly determine the outcome (C, the consequences). In this case, you eat three pieces of apple pie (event A) and it triggered your thoughts, "You're pathetic. You're never going to lose weight. In fact, you're going to be as big as a house come Christmas!" (belief B) which in turn triggered misery and shame (consequence C).

This model applies to more than just thoughts about weight and dieting. I want to make sure you are clear on how it works, so I'm going to walk you through an example that even nondieters can understand.

Scenario 1

Imagine you are driving to work and a car comes out of nowhere and cuts you off. You almost get in a major car accident because of the other driver. You react with immense anger, cursing at the driver, and honking hysterically. Your whole body is tense with anger. When you get to your destination, you continue to carry that anger and you carry it for the entire day. And there you are, being short with your coworkers and easily set off.

Scenario 2

Now let's look at the exact same situation—you are driving to work when a car comes out of nowhere, cuts you off, and almost involves you in a serious motor vehicle accident. This time, instead of reacting with anger, you react with relief. You are feeling tremendously lucky that you weren't in a major car accident. You are overcome with gratitude that nothing major happened. Instead of carrying that anger with you throughout the day, you carry that gratitude, which in turns triggers feeling of appreciation and happiness. You are kind with others and take the initiative to help people around you. You even make a few friendly phone calls to people you haven't spoken to for some time.

These two situations both started with the same activating event (A): another driver cut you off and almost put you in the middle of a major car accident. However, the dominant belief (B) is different in scenario one compared to scenario two. In the former, the belief is that the other driver is horrible and deserves attack. In the latter, the belief is that you are incredibly lucky to have escaped an accident. Because of a difference in your beliefs (B), there is a major difference in the consequences (C) of the "near-miss" accident. On the one hand, consequence one is anger throughout the day while consequence two is deep and lasting gratitude. Night and day, right? And yet they both started with the same activating event (A). This demonstrates clearly that events do not directly cause outcomes. Instead it is our thoughts or beliefs **about** the event that do.

Scenario 1: A—Near accident, B—anger, C—bad mood all day

Scenario 2: A—Near accident, B—relief, C—gratitude all day

This is all good and fine, but I wouldn't be surprised if your response is, "But I don't actually choose what I'm thinking about!" I mean, these thoughts just pop into our heads. They are **automatic**. We're not choosing to curse the other driver or to feel gratitude, it just sort of happens, right? In fact, most of our thoughts throughout the day (thousands of them!) are automatic thoughts—they happen all on their own. For example,

- When the alarm goes off, you think, *Already!?*
- When it's time to go to the gym, you think, *I'm too tired to work out.*
- When your sister calls, you think, *She's going to ask me for a favor, I just know it!*
- When your supervisor walks by, looking serious, you think, *She didn't like the report I prepared!*

These are responses that you don't consciously think through; they are responses that occur automatically. You don't think about it, you don't decide how to respond, the same old thoughts just pop into your head. If that's the case, how do you change your thoughts? How do you control something that is automatic? Well, the first step is becoming aware of your automatic thoughts, and then comming to understand how they influence your emotions and behaviors. Developing this awareness and insight is the focus of the next chapter.

CHAPTER 11

Cognitive Distortions: Automatic Thoughts Gone Wrong

"They always say time changes things, but you actually have to change them yourself."

—ANDY WARHOL

So, we now know that you, like everybody else, have automatic thoughts throughout the day. Automatic thoughts pop into your head all the time, and, much of the time, you're not even fully aware they you're having them. That isn't necessarily a problem because many automatic thoughts are benign. Maybe you're having an automatic thought about what to make for your children's lunch (only to later remember that it is Saturday and they aren't going to school)!

But, and this is another important point, some automatic thoughts are not so benign. These types of automatic thoughts are a result of faulty reasoning. Unfortunately, even if they aren't logical, these thoughts significantly (and negatively) impact how you view your relationships, your potential, and your life in general. The faulty reasoning that generates these unhelpful automatic thoughts are called cognitive distortions.

Psychiatrist Aaron Beck, noted as the father of cognitive-behavioral psychology, developed the concept of cognitive distortions. They are often defined as ways our minds convince us of something that's not really true. These inaccurate thoughts often end up reinforcing negative thinking or emotions.

Cognitive distortions have the power to distort your reality and make you believe things that aren't true, rational, or in keeping with logical thinking. And because actions and decisions are based on these cognitive distortions, they have a lot of influence over how you live your life. Unless you want to live a life based on falsehoods, you will need to take the power away from your distorted, automatic thoughts. The best way to do that is to make these thoughts less and less believable while, at the same time, focusing on an accurate understanding of the situation in front of you.

Let me give you some examples of how cognitive distortions might play out in relation to your diet history.

- Sheila was on a diet when she went to a Thursday night party. Planning to avoid dessert altogether, Sheila instead found herself polishing off three cupcakes. As a result, Sheila tells herself, "Well, I've blown my diet. There is no point going back on the diet now. So, screw it—I'll start again on Monday."

- Patty decides she needs to start working out regularly and plans to go to the gym every day for a month. Two weeks into her fitness routine, Patty accidentally arranges to see a friend at a time that overlaps with her workout time. Unable to find another time, Patty cancels on her friend because Patty didn't want to break her streak of going to the gym every day. And why didn't she want to break that streak? Because Patty was convinced that missing a single day would undo **all** her hard work.

- Claire had lost some weight and was feeling good about herself. While at a party, several people commented on how good she looked. At the same party, Claire runs into an acquaintance she hadn't seen in a while. This person didn't say anything to Claire about how she looks. Claire leaves the party feeling terrible about herself. This blow to her self-esteem comes from Claire's assumption that the acquaintance didn't offer a compliment because Claire didn't look good after all. What about all the other positive comments? Well, to Claire's mind, those people were "just being nice" and didn't really mean what they said.

Do you recognize this type of thinking? Do any of these thoughts sounds familiar to you? Can you relate to having your emotional state dramatically shift based on your own assumptions?

These all-or-nothing thoughts are common among dieters. They are also cognitive distortions, because they don't reflect a rational perspective of reality. Let's examine these thoughts in some depth so you can understand how off the mark they really are.

In the first scenario, Sheila ate off-limits foods and was feeling guilty and discouraged. She also decided that, after having fallen off her diet, she'd stay off until she could get a "fresh start" on Monday. So, why is this irrational? Well, doing a quick calculation, we can estimate that Sheila ate about 1,500 calories more than she had planned. Realistically, that's not a whole lot to undo. But if Sheila goes through the whole weekend with the "I've blown it. I'll start again on Monday" mentality—last-chance eating might drive her to eat an extra 10,000 to 12,000 calories. (As an FYI, last-chance eating is what dieters do in the last few days before they are scheduled to start a new diet. It's their chance to eat as much as possible before they embrace restriction yet again!)

Now, that is a lot more emotional eating to contend with and can lead to more guilt, more discouragement, and needing much more effort to get back to healthy eating. A more logical and rational approach would have been, "I didn't plan for that, but I can return to healthy eating at the next opportunity. There's no reason to wait until after the weekend." Remember, that it's a lot easier to have this rational thought when you're living a diet-free life. Quite simply, there's no drive to eat like crazy when there is no restriction waiting in the wings.

In the second situation, Patty missed an opportunity to spend some time with a friend because Patty couldn't tolerate the thought of not going to the gym every day. In reality, missing one workout out of thirty would not have had a huge effect on her weight, shape, or fitness level. Further, she might have gotten real benefit out of taking time to see a friend. But by seeing things in black-or-white terms—either "I'm sticking to my plan 100 percent" or "I've blown it"—there was no in-between that would have let Patty both stay committed to prioritizing her fitness **and** see a friend when she was available.

In the last situation, Claire was the recipient of several compliments on her appearance. However, Claire completely discounted the positive comments, simply because one person didn't echo them. Claire was selectively ignoring the positive statements that were made and selectively focusing on the neutral encounter. That type of thinking is not logical, because it doesn't take all the data into consideration. And if we were going to take it a step further, the person who didn't compliment Claire was merely not commenting on Claire's appearance. That is socially appropriate behavior that included no judgment of Claire. And yet, Claire viewed it as evidence that the person had a negative view of Claire's appearance.

Claire's interpretation of the interaction reflects another cognitive distortion called "mind reading." Claire decided that she "knew" what the person was thinking when he or she failed to mention her weight loss. But unless Claire has some unique mind-reading talents, the truth is that she doesn't know why the person chose to stay mute about Claire's weight loss.

Looking at all three of these scenarios, it becomes clear that when automatic thoughts are not questioned and are allowed to influence your feelings and actions, you are at risk of acting on distorted information. Preventing this will mean learning how to identify and challenge irrational and often destructive, automatic thoughts.

It is easier to identify your irrational thoughts when you become familiar with the different types of cognitive distortions. As we go through them, make note of which thoughts resonate with you. It is likely that your automatic thoughts include examples of all the following, but there might be three or four types of cognitive distortions that really stand out for you.

All-or-Nothing Thinking

What Is It?

Looking at experiences in absolutes or black-and-white terms. There are no gray areas.

Examples

I am either on a diet 100 percent or not at all.

If I can't make it to the gym every day, there's no point in going at all.

I can never eat French fries if I want to lose weight.

Why It's Distorted

It doesn't account for the value of doing things in moderation. Going to the gym 8 out of 10 days or eating well 80 percent of the time has immense value. All-or-nothing thinking discounts the value of the taking a moderate, sustainable approach to food and exercise.

Overgeneralizing

What Is It?

Viewing a negative event as a pattern of negative events instead of an isolated incident. It often includes words such as "always" or "never."

Examples

I always blow my diet.

I can't stick with anything.

I never stick to my workout plan.

Why It's Distorted

It discounts the times you do things right. In this way, it devalues the positive steps you have taken and overemphasizes the times when you have struggled.

Discounting the Positive

What Is It?

Dismissing compliments or good experiences as being flukes or exceptions.

Examples

I did well this time, but only because I had help.

Yeah, I had a good week but that almost never happens.

He only asked me out because he feels sorry for me.

Why It's Distorted

It denies you the opportunity to feel good about an event or something you've done. It also diminishes the power of positive events to boost your confidence and create momentum—after all, it was just a "fluke" and doesn't really count.

Dwelling on the Negative

What Is It?

Putting extreme emphasis on the negative, while discounting any coexisting positives.

Examples

Yeah, I achieved a goal at the gym today but I still can't do a pull-up. That's what really counts!

Sure, I stuck with my healthy eating plan. But why does that matter, I'm still overweight!

What difference does it make that I'm learning new skills in this program? I still haven't lost 10 pounds!

Why It's Distorted

This thinking makes the negatives significantly more powerful and meaningful than the evidence suggests.

Shoulds/Oughts/Musts

What Is It?

Thinking in terms of "shoulds" without questioning when, who, and why it has been decided that you should do A, B, or C.

Examples

I should always choose the healthiest item on the menu.

I should work out every day.

I should lose 20 pounds before I ask for that promotion.

Why It's Distorted

It's an arbitrary determination based on an extreme idea. This thinking sets you up for failure by establishing unrealistic expectations. It can also deprive you of meaningful experiences by creating arbitrary barriers.

Fortune Telling

What Is It?

Deciding the outcome ahead of time without knowing for certain. Also known as "predicting the future."

Examples

I know I'm not going to eat well, so there's no point in trying.

I know this program isn't going to work for me. I can just tell!

I'll never be slim again. It just isn't in the cards for me.

Why It's Distorted

The future is always an unknown with no guarantees. You don't even acknowledge the possibility of a positive outcome and instead live your life based on "knowing" that your future will be a negative one.

Mind Reading

What Is It?

Mind reading is when you decide you know what another person is thinking, even though they haven't told you themselves. Most often, mind reading results in a negative assumption.

Examples

I know he didn't smile at me because he is disgusted by my weight.

I know she thinks she's better than me, just because she's skinny.

I can tell he doesn't respect me because of my weight. So, no way am I going to talk to him.

Why It's Distorted

It's not possible to know with 100 percent certainty what people are thinking without them telling you. If you are feeling bad about yourself, it is easy to assume that others have negative feelings about you too. But that's an assumption, which might be a distorted version of reality.

Did you recognize your own thinking in that list of cognitive distortions? Are there some distortions that you can relate to more than others? It's common to have a few "favorites." For example, some of my clients spend most of their days trapped in all-or-nothing thinking (and not just about food and weight). Other clients are so discouraged about their weight-loss journey that they consistently predict that they will fail on this program. That's a whole lot of fortune telling going on.

Whatever your faulty thinking looks like, you need to start catching it in the moment. That means catching your distorted thoughts before they have time to influence your decisions and behaviors. Conveniently, the next chapter focuses on just that. In the meantime, below is a summary of cognitive distortions. Reviewing this list will help you understand how automatic thoughts might have contributed to your yoyo dieting throughout the years.

TYPES OF DISTORTIONS			
Cognitive Distortion	WHAT IT IS	WHY IT'S DISTORTED	EXAMPLES
All Or Nothing Thinking	Looking at experiences in absolutes or black and white terms. No gray areas.	Doesn't account for the value in doing things in moderation. Going to the gym at 80% or eating well 80% of the time has immense value. This thinking discredits that.	I am either 100% on my diet or I'm totally off and "cheating" non-stop. If I can't make it to the gym every day, there's no point in going.

TYPES OF DISTORTIONS			
Overgeneral-Izing	Viewing a single negative event as a pattern of negative events. Seeing things as 'always' or 'never'	Overgeneralizing exaggerates the meaning of negative events. It can create a "mountain" out of a "molehill".	I can't stick with anything. I never stick to my work out plans. I always come up with excuses not to go to the gym.
Discounting The Positive	Dismissing compliments or successes as being flukes or exceptions	This type of thinking undervalues positive events. It denies us the opportunity to feel good about something we've done or experienced.	I had a good week but that never usually happens. He only complimented me because his boss was there.
Dwelling On The Negative	Putting extreme emphasis on the negatives so they overshadow the positives.	Makes negative experiences more important and meaningful than they truly are.	I deviated from my plan and ate that cupcake at the party. All my hard word is ruined!

TYPES OF DISTORTIONS			
Shoulds, Oughts, & Musts	Thinking in 'should' terms without questioning why.	It's an arbitrary determination based on an extreme idea. Sets you up for failure with unrealistic expectations.	I should always choose the healthiest menu item. I should exercise every day.
Fortune Telling	Deciding the outcome ahead of time without knowing for certain. Predicting the future.	The future is always an unknown with no guarantees. You don't allow for the possibility of a positive outcome by anticipating a negative one.	I know I'm not going to eat well so there's no point in trying. I'll never lose weight. It just isn't in the cards for me.
Mind Reading	Deciding you know what another person is thinking even though they haven't told you themselves.	It is simply not possible for you to know with 100% certainty what someone else is thinking at any moment.	I know he didn't smile at me because he is disgusted by my weight. I know she thinks she's better than me, just because she's skinny.

CHAPTER 12

Cognitive Distortions Versus Reasonable Responses

"Your mind will answer most questions if you learn to relax and wait for the answer."

—WILLIAM S. BURROUGHS

Now that you know how thinking can become distorted, the next step is to catch these unhealthy thoughts the moment they enter your head. Once you are aware that you are having such thoughts, you can begin the work of debunking them. Yes, it is going to take some getting used to at first because, like most people, you might not be paying attention to the automatic thoughts passing through your head. Even if you do have some awareness of your cognitive distortions, you're likely going to need a lot more awareness to catch them early. And catching them early is vital, because you want to have the time to successfully "talk" yourself out of acting on this irrational thinking.

Changing your thinking is likely to be most relevant when you are struggling with negative emotions, such as anxiety, sadness, loneliness, jealousy, frustration, anger, guilt, low self-esteem, despair, worry, boredom, and fatigue. You will likely have noticed that it is generally when you are experiencing emotions like those that your cognitive distortions come out in full force. For this reason, one of the best ways of training yourself to identify distorted thinking in the moment is to pay close attention to your thinking when you are having distressing emotions. So be on the lookout! The next time you feel an uncomfortable emotion, start asking yourself what you are thinking. In this way, you are likely to come face to face with some of your cognitive distortions.

To make this process easier to learn, I'm providing a tool I call a "thought tracker." This is a worksheet that you will use to (a) track your cognitive distortions, and (b) come up with alternate rational, logical thoughts. These are often called reasonable responses. To ensure that you are comfortable using this worksheet, let me share an example of how to put this tool to use.

Let's say it's a rainy, dreary Thursday evening. You have just gotten home from work, and, out of habit, you grab a bag of chips and start snacking. It doesn't take long for you to realize that you're experiencing some distressing emotions: guilt, shame, and frustration all rolled into one. As soon as you become aware of these emotions, you stop everything you are doing long enough to ask yourself, "What thoughts are going through my head right now?"

On this particular Thursday evening, you realize that most of your thoughts are about an incident where you made a mistake at work. The dominant thoughts in your head are, *I'm always screwing everything up, Everyone thinks I'm terrible at my job, and I never do anything right.* These thoughts are triggering your real negative emotions and yet each one of them is a cognitive distortion. In fact, that triad of thoughts is a classic example of overgeneralizing, dwelling on the negative, and all-or-nothing thinking. In other words, your thoughts don't accurately reflect reality. (Although, until you learn to challenge them, they still have the power to effectively trigger unhelpful emotions and problematic behaviors.)

Having identified the cognitive distortions that are unduly influencing your emotions, the next step is to replace them with a more reasonable and rational response. Instead of thinking, *I'm always screwing everything up,* a more reasonable response might be, *I made a mistake, but it was one that anyone could have made in the same situation.* Instead of thinking, *Everyone thinks I'm terrible at my job,* a more reasonable response might be, *I do a lot of things well at work—no one is judging me for one simple mistake.* And, instead of thinking, *I never do anything right,* a more reasonable response might be, *I do a lot of things right. I just made one simple mistake. It doesn't define me.*

Is this starting to make a little bit more sense? Just to make sure it is really hitting home, let's look at a week of thought tracking from one of my actual clients.

DATE	SITUATION	THOUGHT	REASONABLE RESPONSE
7/14	Luncheon with co-workers.	They are all thinner than me. I'll never get there!	I'm getting closer every day. I'm focusing on being a better me and not comparing myself.
7/14	Watching TV. Bored.	I want to eat. A few chips won't matter.	I'm not hungry. I want to learn to eat when I'm hungry, not when I'm bored.
7/15	End of the night. Craving Ice cream.	I've had a great week. I deserve to treat myself with ice cream.	I have had a great week and I deserve to continue feeling good about myself. If I'm not hungry, I can treat myself with something other than food.

DATE	SITUATION	THOUGHT	REASONABLE RESPONSE
7/17	Out to dinner with friends.	Everything looks so good- I want to eat all the bad stuff! I can make up for it at the gym tomorrow.	There is no "bad stuff" anymore. I can have anything I want when I'm hungry. I don't use exercise to "make up" for eating anymore. I use it to feel healthy and to have fun.
7/18	Home with no plans.	Eating everything in the fridge will make me feel better.	I'm just bored and food is not the answer for boredom. I can do a million other things. I'll start by taking a walk.
7/18	Can't sleep.	Eating is the best way to distract myself when I can't sleep.	I NEVER feel good when I eat late at night. I want to do what makes me feel good.
7/19	Just got home from brunch.	I totally blew my diet by eating WAY too much.	I'm not on a diet. This is a way of life so I can't "blow" it. One large meal is no big deal. I will just refocus on eating healthy now.

I hope this example has helped you truly understand how this works. In a nutshell, you are paying attention to your thoughts and replacing the distorted views with reasonable alternatives. You're doing this work because distorted thoughts often play a big role in keeping the yoyo diet cycle going.

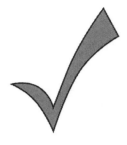 **Take Action:** Now it's your turn. Use the worksheet to track your distorted thoughts and to start building a collection of reasonable responses. I've provided an example as a running start. Remember, the more you track your thoughts, the easier it will get. Don't worry if the same cognitive distortions and reasonable responses come up again and again on your worksheet. This just means you are getting more practice and will be able to access your reasonable thoughts when you truly need them. (For example, in the middle of a binge driven by all-or-nothing thinking).

Some days you will have more distorted thinking than others. That is completely natural –just be prepared to take some time to track your thoughts when the irrational views start to surface. You often won't get much warning before your distorted, automatic thoughts kick in. I've provided an example on the worksheet to help get you going.

THOUGHT TRACKER			
DATE	SITUATION	DISTORTED THOUGHT	REASONABLE RESPONSE
7/14	Got home from work and started snacking on chips	I always screw everything up!	I made one mistake, but I do a lot of things well!

CHAPTER 13

Power Thoughts: Helping to Keep Cognitive Distortions at Bay

"The most powerful relationship you will ever have is the relationship with yourself."

—STEVE MARABOLI

Do you remember the illustrated children's book, *The Little Engine That Could?* Well, if you don't, it was about a small train engine that kept saying "I think I can, I think I can . . ." to get itself up and over the mountain. The little blue engine was talking with strength and conviction, and ultimately this created strength and conviction within the little locomotive. The engine wasn't lying to itself, it wasn't telling fairytales, it was simply telling the truth. It was just a truth that it had not previously embraced.

This is exactly what *power thoughts* are. They are ways to talk to yourself with strength and conviction, which then helps bring your own strength and conviction to the surface. Power thoughts are like those supportive, helpful, gut feelings that you know to be true but which you ignore due to those pesky (and sometimes, downright nasty) distortions.

Finding your personal power thoughts is definitely worth the time and effort required. But after years of burying them under all-or-nothing thinking and other distortions, how exactly should you go about unearthing them? Hopefully, by this point in the program, you have accumulated a whole boatload of reasonable responses on your thought trackers. And, conveniently enough, within that pile of reasonable responses are your power thoughts. You might need to flesh them out, but the bones of your power thoughts are ready and waiting on your thought tracker sheets.

Your power thoughts are the responses that encourage you, that you can connect with, and which take into account both logical thinking and healthy emotions. They probably aren't the thoughts that come into your head automatically, but that doesn't mean they don't belong front and center. In fact, you want them right where you can access them again and again. That's because they are the thoughts that make you feel empowered, and make you say "Hell, yeah, I can do this!" They are also the thoughts you truly buy into and believe wholeheartedly. Looking at some examples together should help make sure the concept of power thoughts is clear.

Let's say you are extremely prone to all-or-nothing thinking. As a result, the thought, "I need to stick to my healthy eating plan 100 percent or not at all," takes up a lot of your headspace. Perhaps you've had a lot of reasonable responses to this type of thinking during the past couple of weeks, but the one that truly speaks to you is this: "I will have the most success managing my weight by not being too rigid and using the 80/20 approach." If that's the response that speaks to you above all the others, then that is one of your power thoughts.

Ready for another example? Okay, let's pretend you're the queen-of-dwelling-on-the-negative, (and for some of you, that probably isn't much of a stretch)! After a long day at work, you're left with thoughts like *I did a decent job, but I didn't do it fast enough,* and *My supervisor was happy with my work, but I know it wasn't as good as it could have been.*

Luckily, having used your thought tracker, you now have reasonable responses, one of which might end up being your next power thought. Will it be, *It was more than I did the day before,* or *Any effort I put in is worthwhile?* Or maybe the thought, *Every effort I make that is more than nothing gives me value and is worthy of recognition,* is the one that really speaks you. Whichever thought(s) leaves you feeling upbeat, optimistic, and well, powerful, *and* which you wholeheartedly believe, has hereby earned the title of power thought.

If "should" statements are a regular part of your thinking, thoughts like, *I shouldn't focus so much on myself,* or *I should use my day off to help others,* might be circulating through your brain on a regular basis. Having learned how to counter those cognitive distortions, you now have in front of you a list of reasonable responses that includes, *It's important to focus on myself in addition to others,* and *It's not selfish to take care of me.* Maybe out of all the reasonable responses on the list, the one that speaks to you the loudest is, *I need to take care of myself first, if I am going to take care of others.* Again, if this thought is something you truly believe and it makes you feel strong *and* empowered, then you have another power thought on your hands.

If you are still unsure about which of your statements are power thoughts, here's another approach. Compile your reasonable responses on one sheet of paper. (At the end of this chapter, you'll find a "My Power Thoughts" worksheet that you can use for this purpose.) All you need to do is transcribe the reasonable responses from your "Thought Tracker" worksheet onto this new worksheet. Don't worry about transcribing anything else from the Thought Tracker worksheet—you will only be looking at your reasonable responses. Once you have them all written on the "My Power Thoughts" worksheet (use several copies of the worksheet, if needed), read through the list. While you read, keep the following questions in mind:

1. Are there any responses that just feel amazing when you read them? They make you want to say, "Damn right!" or "I am awesome!"

2. Do you notice any repetition in these responses? Are there any common themes that come up repeatedly in your collection of reasonable responses?

3. Are there any responses that you know in your heart are true and yet you struggle to say them confidently and out loud?

Next, circle the statements on your worksheet that lead you to answer yes to any of the above questions. To help you with this process, let's go through each question separately. For the first question, the thoughts that make you feel great when you read them and sound like they are perfect! You can keep them just as they are and transcribe them "as is" on your "good copy" of the "My Power Thoughts" worksheet.

In response to the second question, you have identified multiple responses that seem to reflect the same theme. Can you combine them into one or two power thoughts? For example, perhaps a lot of your cognitive distortions revolve around feeling left out. You might have reworked those thoughts into a collection of reasonable responses along these lines.

I know I'm well-liked. I have a lot of friends who enjoy being around me.

> *My friends and I always have a good time when we get together.*
>
> *I've had many friends for a long time.*
>
> *I know that my friends and I are busy. It's natural that we don't always have time for one another.*

A power thought that combines these statements might look like this.

> *I'm well liked. I have lots of friends, and I know they enjoy spending time with me.*

It's simple, powerful, true, but it's also concise. By combining several reasonable responses into one powerful statement, you will have created what I like to call an "ultra" power thought!

After considering the third question, you identified reasonable responses that you struggle to say with conviction. Take some time to think about those responses for a little longer. If you know in your heart of hearts that they are true, and yet still have trouble verbalizing these statements, it is likely that you are hitting on some of your core issues. What does that mean for this exercise? It means that although the statements have immense value, they might be too much, too soon. In other words, they are so far removed from your negative, automatic thoughts that you are having difficulty embracing them for the moment. So, go for the soft sell.

Look at these responses and see if there is a way you can tweak or adjust them to make them more palatable for right now. For example, your reasonable response might be, *I am beautiful and the most important person in my own life. I deserve self-love and self-care.* This is a powerful thought and absolutely true, but if it's a new thought to you, it might be hard to embrace just yet.

Instead, a similar, but lower-key, statement might be easier to get fully behind without any reservations. How about this: *I am important and deserving of self-love and self-care.* This statement is still true and still powerful, but it also doesn't trigger any resistance to adopting it as one of your power thoughts. This technique allows you to gradually introduce "ultra" power thoughts by toning them down. Once you're comfortable with the "lighter" version, you can introduce the more powerful version of this reasonable response to your list of power thoughts.

Take Action: You have your work cut out for you at this point. You need to get working on identifying the power thoughts that speak to you, drive you, empower you, and to which you have a strong connection. Your power thoughts play an important role in breaking free from yoyo dieting, so the sooner you get working on identifying them, the better!

You might have two. You might have 200. There is no correct number—as long as they meet the criteria listed earlier, they're good to go. So good to go in fact, that you can put them down on your "My Power Thoughts" worksheet and start reviewing them regularly.

Putting Your Power Thoughts to Work

Take Action: Once you've got your power thoughts picked out and written down, I strongly encourage you to put them in places where they'll be most effective. In other words, put them in places that allow the statements to do their part in offsetting the automatic thoughts that keep you stuck in old patterns.

Let me give you a few examples of what I mean by that.

You're feeling some unpleasant combination of bad and "snack-y" while watching television. In a situation like that, keep your power thoughts on your couch or coffee table near the TV. This makes it easy for you to review them in an effort to counteract automatic thoughts, like *Eating a big bowl of ice cream with lots of chocolate sauce is the only thing that will make me feel better.*

If it's your ten o'clock coffee break at work, that is likely to find you using chocolate chip cookies to manage project anxiety, then better make sure you have your power thoughts close at hand. Maybe a sticky note on your desk? A few power thoughts strategically placed on your bulletin board? Whatever works for you!

If it's bedtime when your automatic, *I have to go on a diet because I'm so fat* thoughts start swirling around your head, then have a handy, dandy copy of your power thoughts on your bedside table.

Think about when and where you are most likely to need your power thoughts, and make a plan to have them readily accessible. I've had clients who have written their power thoughts on index cards and kept a stack in their purse or briefcase for moments of need. I had another client who laminated a page of power thoughts and kept it handy. Here's the bottom line: You want to make it easy to repeat your power thoughts over and over again. The eventual goal is to have these power thoughts push your longstanding cognitive distortions aside. Then, these power thoughts can take over as your new (and healthy) automatic thoughts.

My Power Thoughts

1. _____
   _____

2. _____
   _____

3. _____
   _____

4. _____
   _____

5. _____
   _____

6. _____
   _____

7. _____
   _____

8. _____
   _____

9. _____
   _____

10. _____
    _____

Change Your Life

CHAPTER 14

The Power of Habits

"Though no one can go back and make a brand new start, anyone can start from now and make a brand new ending."

—CARL BARD

So far, we have talked about focus, and we have talked about thoughts—the missing ingredient in this model is behavior, or action. Changing your focus has hopefully given you a renewed sense of purpose, some true motivation that you connect with at your core, and a new approach to achieving your goals. Changing your thinking should have challenged some of the unhealthy thoughts that have been getting in your way for so many years. It should also have helped you generate rational and empowering thoughts that truly resonate with you.

When I first started to change my focus and my thoughts, I felt empowered and motivated. I was so proud of myself and felt like I could take on the world. But, then, disaster struck—I went on a business trip, and the progress I made began to unravel quickly. It was a real doozy of a business trip in terms of my eating and thinking. It felt like "game over"! It was as if everything I had learned and built within myself was completely lost. I seemed to fall into old habits without giving it a second thought. It felt like I was on automatic pilot, and all that work I had done to change my focus and my thoughts wasn't making one iota of a difference.

Of course, that wasn't true. (In fact, it would be fair to call that "discounting the positive"—a familiar face from our chapter on cognitive distortions.) I was just running into a scenario I had not prepared for and old habits naturally took over. On every business trip before this, I would eat every meal out, I would load up at breakfast buffets, and choose the most indulgent items on the menu for lunch and dinner. I wouldn't exercise, I would sleep late, and I would "forget" to meditate. It could be summed up simply: me not taking good care of myself. This time around, it also involved not taking the time to challenge my old thinking and my old behaviors. That left plenty of room for old habits to drop by for an (unwanted) visit!

Habits are all about behavioral change. And after you've completed the first three sections of this book, a big part of what will get in the way of ending the yoyo cycle for good is leftover bad habits. That's the bad news. The good news is that every habit can be changed!

Statistically speaking, it takes 66 days to create a new habit. That might sound like a lot, but what that also means is it takes 66 days to break a habit. That's incredible when you think you have been doing something one way for your entire life and it only takes 66 days to stop that habit! It also means it takes 66 days before something is truly automated and habitual—meaning you do it without thinking. But it takes considerably less time for it to get easier and more comfortable.

A little public service announcement: Remember that 66 days is the average. For some people, a new habit might take fewer than 66 days to be fully established. For others, it might take longer. Also, different habits might be easier or harder to fully embrace. So, whatever you do, don't panic if at day 66 you're still finding it hard to not finish everything on your plate when you're no longer hungry. Maybe this is a case of needing 72 or 83 days. However long it takes, it'll be a lot less than the years you've lost developing the yoyo diet habit.

Hopefully, the following example will make it even easier to understand the importance of changing automatic behaviors (habits). I had a client, named Bea, who worked from home every afternoon from 2:00 p.m. to 6:00 p.m. The primary problem that brought Bea to my office was that even though she could work right through dinner without feeling hungry, almost every night around 10:00 p.m., a full-fledged, binge-eating episode would kick in.

When Bea and I went through her usual daily routine, it became clear that she had some long -standing eating habits that might explain some of her problems. Every day at 2:00 p.m., Bea would set up to work on the bar counter in her kitchen. While working away during the next four hours, Bea was also eating away. Eating away for the entire time, it turned out. Bea would snack on chips, fruit, cookies, whatever was within arm's reach. The amazing part was that Bea barely realized she was doing it! It wasn't unusual for food to be on the counter, and it wasn't unusual for Bea to work at the bar in her kitchen.

Combine that with four hours of eating that was entirely mindless (just automatic hand to food, hand to mouth) and Bea wasn't even conscious of her own eating behavior. Sure, Bea could have told you that she ate a handful of this or a handful of that every now and then, but she would have vehemently denied that she was eating thousands of calories during that four-hour period. Bea didn't realize the extent of her mindless eating until she started to track it. Once she did, Bea knew she had to change her routine.

Working together, we decided that Bea moving to another part of the house to work was the best solution. Proceeding with that plan, Bea set up a little office space for herself in the guest room. Despite her good intentions, and even after the office move, Bea found herself spending a lot of time thinking about food during her 2:00 to 6:00 p.m. witching hour. She was snacking significantly less, but she was still thinking a lot about food.

As a next step, we focused on ensuring that Bea ate a satisfying lunch before sitting down to work. Still, Bea's thoughts centered around food while she was working. Clearly, Bea had created a habit. It was no longer about hunger or satiation. It was just something she did during that time of the day, and it was also something she had been doing for years. Now came the hard, albeit temporary, part. Bea simply had to push through and not allow herself to eat mindlessly during her working hours. If she was authentically hungry, fine. But if it was a case of eating for fun, for comfort, or to pass the time, that was not part of the lifestyle Bea wanted to create.

I won't pretend that making this change was a breeze for Bea. In fact, the first week was super tough! But Bea made it through the tough days, and she found that the second week was significantly easier. By the third week, Bea still had to keep an eye on her urges to snack, but she really didn't find it difficult to not act on her occasional urge. Eventually (right about 66 days in), working without mindless eating had become a habit for Bea. Even before the magic 66 day, Bea's new daily routine got easier and easier to follow. Even better, because Bea wasn't eating mindlessly for four hours a day, she was hungry at dinnertime. In turn, eating at mealtime kept Bea from finding herself ravenous and craving high-calorie food (and lots of it) just as the clock struck 11:00 p.m.

Sometimes people get scared of the work needed to change old habits. They remember sayings like, "Old habits die hard." and "You can't teach an old dog new tricks." But, those sayings are good examples of "fortune telling"—predicting and putting a negative spin on the future. Don't let a cognitive distortion scare you away from embarking on this habit-change process.

This step is so important to finally "Shattering the Yoyo" that the trying, the failing, and the trying again on the way to success will pay off eventually. I know this, because I've seen it happen time and time again. I have had many clients who have been diehard dieters with a whole host of unhealthy automatic behaviors (habits) for years. And yet, they were able to break bad habits and build new, healthy ones, as they moved toward weight-management success.

CHAPTER 15

Know Thy Enemy: Identify Your Danger Zones

*"You are imperfect, permanently and inevitably flawed.
And you are beautiful."*

—AMY BLOOM

The *danger zone*—maybe this is a term you associate with singer Kenny Loggins from the 1980s or with the animated television series, *Archer*. But if you are an experienced yoyo dieter, chances are that you have a different understanding of this term. For dieters, a danger zone is a situation that triggers them to feel unable to control their urges, cravings, and behaviors.

It is a circumstance in which you are at significant risk of bingeing, grazing, eating for emotional reasons, or mindlessly munching away. Before I overcame my eating and weight problems by using this program, travel was one of my danger zones. You might be aware of your danger zones. But, if you aren't, there are ways to figure out when and where you are most vulnerable to eating in a way that doesn't support your emotional or physical health.

To get you thinking about your own personal danger zones, here is a list of situations that many dieters find challenging.

- Restaurant eating
- Social events
- Business meals
- Being home alone
- Food "pushers" and/or family pressure
- Boredom
- TV watching/snacking
- Transitioning from work to home
- Work stress
- Traveling
- Buffets/parties
- Snacking at work
- Too tired, lazy, stressed to cook
- Junk food around the house
- Sensory cravers
- Late-night snacking
- Reward eating ("I deserve a treat.")
- "I'm so tired!" eating

These are just some examples of situation that might be danger zones for you. If they are danger zones, then your eating is usually mindless, excessive, and/are frantic when encountered. Danger zones trigger eating that essentially has nothing to do with hunger. It might have to do with emotions, fatigue, habit, or pressure from others, but it isn't about providing your body with the food it needs.

Recognizing your danger zones and developing a corresponding action plan (don't worry, I'll explain action plans in the next chapter) is important to the success of this program. For that reason, we're going to take the time right here, right now, to review potential danger zones in more detail. Remember to take note of the situations that apply to you—that information is going to come in handy when you start working on your action plans.

> **Restaurant eating**—Some people have been dieting for so long that they are used to keeping their kitchen full of healthy foods and devoid of junk food. If that's you, you shop regularly, choose food that you won't binge on, and make sure that healthy snacks, not cookies and chips, are available at a moment's notice. But when restaurants are a danger zone, as soon as you walk through the door, the gloves come off. Everything you know about healthy eating goes out the window. Instead, you make the most of the opportunity to eat "bad" food, and lots of it!

> That could mean ordering an appetizer (or two), a main meal, and a dessert, even though you stopped being physically hungry halfway through the entrée. It might mean ordering foods that are off-limits, like a jumbo platter of deep-fried anything or polishing off everybody's leftovers, just because they are there. If you recognize yourself in this description, then restaurant eating belongs on your list of danger zones. To be perfectly clear, the fact that it is a challenging eating situation for you doesn't mean it's now a no-no. That would be all-or-nothing diet thinking. It just means that you need to be particularly mindful when you are going out for breakfast, lunch, or dinner.

> **Social events**—It's no surprise that social events are a danger zone for some people, because this situation overlaps with restaurant eating. Suddenly, you are given access to foods that might never cross the door of your own home (having been banished because they are

too "fattening" or off-limits). Just as for the restaurant example, at a social event, it is possible to turn your eating habits 180 degrees in the opposite direction. This can happen at all sorts of get-togethers: business events, potlucks, holidays, or parties. You name it, if there's a social event that includes food, it's possible to eat far too much, because, being out of your own element, your goals and guidelines seem so distant. Is this one of your danger zones?

➤ **Business meals**—Business meals can include some specific challenges. The timing must work for everyone, rather than meeting the needs of your physical hunger (or lack thereof). The location of the meal is often outside your control. You might find yourself at a place that offers a whole lot of off-limits foods and not much else. There's nothing wrong with that, if that's what you're in the mood for. But if you're still adjusting to giving yourself permission to eat high-fat/high-calorie food, being put in a position of having that be your only choice, opens the door to I've blown it—I might as well binge diet thinking. Of course, as you progress in this program, you'll navigate such situation in a much healthier way, but in the early stages of this program, business meals might remain a danger zone.

Complicating the practical considerations, are the social pressures that can raise their ugly heads during business meals. For example, maybe it's expected that you indulge just like everyone else, even if you truly have a hankering for salad and chicken. I've known many businesswomen who have working dinners with businessmen and find themselves feeling pressured to order more than a salad. It's as if they are expected to jump on the "gigantic bowl of pasta" or "steak and all the fixing" bandwagon even if that wouldn't respect their authentic wants and (bodily) needs.

➢ **Being home alone**—For some people, being home alone is the ultimate danger zone. This is likely to apply to anyone who hides their eating from others. The shame and guilt you associate with eating keeps you from eating much of anything in public. But as soon as you are set loose in your own home, all bets are off. This is particularly true if you have undereaten while out with others. Now, your physical hunger has grown so strong that any thought of eating in a relaxed and mindful manner flew out the window a long time ago. As you learn to trade your negative feelings about eating for life-affirming power thoughts, you will be able to eat anywhere and anytime without embarrassment. That will be the first step in changing your home from a danger zone to a place of peace and relaxation.

➢ **Food "pushers" and/or family pressure**—Are you familiar with the concept of food pushers? They would be the people in your life who are constantly pushing food on you and taking great offense if you politely decline their offer. For many people, the food pushers in their lives are family members—parents, grandparents, in-laws, even siblings. Sometimes, it is a friend or a spouse/boyfriend/girlfriend who feels threatened by the work you are doing to manage your weight. Whoever it is for you, if you know that it makes these people happy to see you eat, it can be hard to turn down the cupcake, cookies, or sandwich they are offering. And sometimes, even if you muster the strength to say, "No," "No," and "No" again, they have no intention of stopping their food pushing! If you have a food pusher in your life, then a visit with them is likely a serious danger zone.

➢ **Boredom—**Boredom is just one of the emotions that can also be a danger zone. This danger zone is usually the strongest when you are at home alone. But unlike the earlier "at home" danger zone that was all about escaping the prying eyes of others and eating (bingeing) in peace, this danger zone is about mindless eating. It is something you do when your brain or body are not occupied or fulfilled. I'm willing to guess that if you're a boredom eater, a lot of this eating happens in front of the television or the computer. What you have then is mindless and distracted eating that leads to eating a lot of food. Often, you won't even be truly conscious of the fact that you have polished off a pint of ice cream, a dozen cookies, and a plate full of crackers and cheese. Not a great situation when you are trying to develop healthy eating patterns. If this is your danger zone, you are definitely in good company!

➢ **TV watching/snacking—**This danger zone overlaps a lot with boredom eating. The only difference is that in this case it isn't about being bored. In fact, you might be quite captivated by what you are watching on TV. Instead, this danger zone is about eating simply because you associate screen time with eating time. It's now a full-blown habit for you to sit down with the remote control in one hand and an ice cream sandwich in the other. Sometimes it isn't just the screen that triggers an I-need-to-eat-right-now response. Sometimes it's a certain chair that you associate with snacking or a certain time of day that just happens to coincide with the time of day when all the "good shows" are on. Whatever the trigger is, the end result is the same: You've entered a danger zone where your eating is about habit, not about mindfully nourishing yourself.

➢ **Transitioning from work to home—**Sometime a danger zone is not about a place, it's about a time of day. If it's been a long day at the office, it makes sense that you need some "transition time" between when you walk in your front door and when you have settled into life at home. For a lot of people, this transition time has become all about absentmindedly going through the refrigerator or cupboards looking for food. In most cases, it is not done out of hunger but out of habit. (If it is out of hunger, consider bringing an extra snack with you to work. Letting yourself get so hungry that you need to start foraging for food the moment you get home is not part of this program!) It's also possible that because the kitchen is a central location in most houses, being there immediately after work is all that it takes to trigger a hunt for food.

> **Work stress**—Work stress can put you into the danger zone in many ways. For some of you, work stress keeps you so busy and overwhelmed that you simply forget to eat. Then, several hours after you first realized you were hungry, you find yourself "starving." The next thing you know, you are eating your way through a pile of food much bigger than what would have satisfied you, had you eaten earlier. Or, maybe you use food to cope with or distract yourself from stress at work. You might be the type who uses sweet, dessert-y foods in response to work stress. Or, maybe it's all about chips, pretzels, and anything salty and crunchy that you can find in your desk or in the breakroom. In both cases, food is being used to meet an emotional need ("I need something to get me through this work load!") rather than a physical need for food.

> **Traveling**—Remember the story I shared about losing sight of this program while I was on a business trip. Well, that's because traveling is a serious danger zone for me. If you're anything like I was, you're generally a healthy eater. You

take good care of yourself; are mindful of what, why, and where you are eating; and you've successfully introduced this program to your everyday life. But, as soon as you go on a trip or vacation, everything changes. Sometimes this is because so many factors are out of your control (for example, your sleep pattern, your schedule, your ability to shop for groceries and make your own meals). Feeling overwhelmed, you simply say, "screw it," and give yourself permission to eat everything and anything "just because" or, feeling frustrated, you binge to sooth that emotion (temporarily, of course, temporarily)! In this way, traveling provides an excuse for bingeing until you get back home and into your familiar environment.

➢ **Buffets/parties**—This type of danger zone is driven by a need to make the most of a buffet or free food. I mean, who doesn't want to get their money's worth? And free food, well, even better! So, there you are at the free wine and cheese event, filling and refilling your glass and your plate. The focus on getting a bargain gets in the way of staying connected with your goal to be a healthy, natural eater (not a get-while-the-getting-is-good eater). Know this, if free food is one of your danger zones, you're not alone. The deprivation that is part and parcel of dieting makes "free" food (and often free, off-limits food) hard to ignore.

➢ **Snacking at work**—Do you work in an office that has a breakroom that is filled to the brim with snacks? Is it doughnut Monday and cookies Friday at your workplace? Then there's the staff member with the "help yourself" policy when it comes to the candy jar on her desk. The possibilities are endless. The combination of free food and opportunity make (over)snacking at work a common problem. That the food is so accessible, just adds to the temptation. I mean, if you had to walk a couple of blocks to get a cookie, chances are you'd think twice about doing it. But, if all you have to do is walk down the hallway, well, that's a whole other ball of wax. And that's why workplace = danger zone for a whole lot of people.

> **Too tired, lazy, stressed to cook**—Ever notice that when you put energy and effort into food prep and making homecooked meals, your eating takes a sharp turn toward wonderful and nutritious? And that you feel great after a homecooked meal? Other times, you're too tired, too lazy, or too darn stressed to imagine embarking on a homemade black bean soup adventure. Instead, you load up on cheese quesadillas that aren't even that good. That's a familiar story.

Many people can eat delicious, yet healthy, food when they put aside time for cutting up the onions, carrots, and celery that bring so much flavor to homemade soup (or chili, or spaghetti sauce). But when food prep drops off the schedule, quick and easy (and often too much of quick and easy!) becomes the meal plan. If time management and fatigue are a constant struggle for you, there is a good chance that this is one of your danger zones.

> **Junk food around the house**—Easy access to comfort food or junk food increases the chances that you'll grab a handful in response to habit, stress, or whatever reason justifies an extra-large bowl of Ben and Jerry's ice cream at that particular moment. Sometimes, you're not even the one who brought the danger zone into the house. In fact, you might be stocking the fridge with fruits and vegetables and the cupboards with brown rice and almond butter. But, your significant other was jonesing for cookies

and chips, and suddenly there they are, front and center on your kitchen counter.

After years of dieting, it is common to slip back into obsessing about off-limits foods. When they're in the house, it isn't hard to move from obsessing about them to eating vast amounts of them. The same can be said about "special occasion" foods, like your leftover birthday cake or all that Halloween candy you bought just in case you were visited by hundreds of kids. Take heart, there will come a time when dieting is a distant memory and obsessional thinking about food will also be a thing of the past. But until that time, having formerly off-limits foods in the house can be a danger zone. (It doesn't mean they should be banned, just that you need an action plan to manage your urges.)

➤ **Sensory cravers**—If you are a sensory craver, temptation can be triggered by seeing, smelling, or otherwise sensing food that you consider particularly yummy or off-limits. Have you ever watched a television commercial for something (for example, pizza, a Snickers bar, potato chips) and been so obsessed with that item that you "had to" go out and get it? Have you ever walked past a shop and had the smell of food consume you to the point that you just couldn't get it out of your head? (Hello, Cinnabon. I'm talking to you!). This can be one of your danger zones, even if you are generally able to plan your meals and stick with the plan. Such is the power of the senses to invoke strong, unrelenting cravings.

➤ **Late-night snacking**—Are you the type of person who eats fairly healthy during the day, but once night hits, well, it's a whole different story? There can be different reasons for this late-night "snack attack," including going too long without eating, fear of hunger (a common "scar" of dieting), a need for self-soothing, or an antidote for boredom. Most of these reasons for eating a lot at night are not about physical hunger but about how food has become the answer to emotional needs. By following the Shatter the Yoyo program, you'll find more appropriate answers for those needs. You will learn how crucial it is to not let yourself get overly hungry. Until you have mastered those steps, it might be that nighttime snacking will continue to be one of your danger zones.

> **Reward eating ("I deserve a treat.")**—The fact is that eating causes all sorts of chemical reactions, including the release of hormones that leave you feeling happier, calmer, and well, rewarded. So, it shouldn't be too much of a surprise that food as a reward is a universal phenomenon. Kids who do their homework, get dessert. You finish your last exam, and you're going out for wings! As we get older and find our days full of "to-dos," it can feel like the only reward you have time for is the extra-large, chocolate fudge sundae that you stop for on your way home from work. Of course, it does feel rewarding for a minute or two. And, it's that minute or two that keeps you hooked— not unlike a gambler's high. Until you find some other way to acknowledge the work you do, celebrate happy events, and reward yourself for just getting through a busy day, reward eating is likely to remain a danger zone.

> **"I'm-so-tired!" eating**—This is the danger zone that comes knocking when you are tired to the bone. Maybe you're trying to complete a report by pulling an all-nighter, but the next thing you know you've made and eaten a pot of mac and cheese. ("Did I really just do that?!") Or all those middle-of-the-night interruptions to feed the baby leave you grazing all day just to keep yourself from

falling asleep before noon. This is a danger zone that has a real biological basis. As we've already seen, not enough sleep makes your appetite hormones go haywire and your cravings for high-calorie foods go through the roof.

This list of danger zones is not exhaustive, but it does include the most common challenges that I have run into during my years of working with chronic dieters. You might have other danger zones that are not on this list and that doesn't make them any less important. The important thing is being aware, because out of awareness will come your action plans.

As I said earlier, some of you might be well aware of your danger zones. If you're still uncertain after reviewing the list in this chapter, there's another approach to uncovering your danger zones. It requires you to track your eating for a couple of weeks. I'm not suggesting food logging as a way of controlling your eating (some diet programs use food logs that way—the idea being if you have to write it down, you might not eat it).

The purpose of the food log I'm suggesting is solely data gathering. For that reason, weights and measurements are not necessary. No recording how many ounces of this or cups of that you've eaten. You also don't have to estimate if the chicken you ate was the size or your palm, or list the number of calories in the chocolate chip cookie that kept you company at coffee break.

You simply want to record what you ate, at what time, and what else was going on emotionally, socially, and physically, at that time. Entries might make mention of your mother-in-law's health, feeling bored, or being surrounded by "free food." An example of a day's food log might look something like this.

TIME	FOOD	NOTES
7:00 am	Coffee and a breakfast sandwich from Starbucks	Rushing to work.
10:00 am	Yogurt	Brought from home.
1:00 pm	Steak sandwich, fries, bread and butter	Lunch out with clients.
4:00 pm	A few small candies	From receptionist's desk.
7:00 pm	Chips and salsa	Home. Not very hungry.
10:15 pm	2 bowls of cereal	Felt super hungry before going to bed.

As you can see—the serving sizes are not what's important here. What's important is what you ate due to hunger, what you ate due to your schedule, and what you ate for a variety of other reasons (for example, boredom, sadness, fatigue). Looking at the food log sample above, do you have any initial hunches about this person's danger zones? Business eating could be an issue (large lunch with clients), as could be freebies (the candy from the receptionist's desk), and late-night snacking (cereal before bed). But, this is just one day. We would need to look at a couple of weeks to identify meaningful trends. Let me give an example of what a food log might look like during a longer period of time. Here is Lauren's food log for an entire week.

TIME	FOOD	NOTES
Mon 7:30 am	Protein Bar	N/A
10:30 am	Yogurt and granola	Food prepped for the week!
12:30 pm	Salad with chicken breast	
4:00 pm	Apple and peanut butter	
7:30 pm	Fish filet with green beans and asparagus	
10:30 pm	2 plates of crackers and cheese	Dinner didn't satisfy me for very long. Tried to avoid eating but finally went for the crackers and cheese.
Tues 7:30 am	Protein bar	
10:30 am	Yogurt and granola	
12:30 pm	Salad with chicken breast	
3:30 pm	2 handfuls trail mix	
4:00 pm	Bag of chips from the breakroom	Boss asked me to stay an extra hour to get project done. I agreed even though I really wanted to go home!
6:30 pm	Steak with creamed spinach	
Weds 7:30 am	Protein bar	
10:30 am	Yogurt and granola	

TIME	FOOD	NOTES
12:30 pm	Sandwich- turkey, lettuce, sprouts, tomato, mustard, avocado	
3:00 pm	Jumbo chocolate chip muffin	Forgot to pack a snack. Was hungry and bought the first yummy thing I saw.
7:00 pm	Bread and olive oil, some fried calamari, fettuccini alfredo, tiramisu, wine	Girls night out. Ate so much I felt a little uncomfortable by the time the evening was over.
Thurs 7:30 am	Protein bar	
10:30 am	Yogurt and granola	
12:30 pm	Salad with chicken	
3:30 pm	Apple and peanut Butter	
7:15 pm	Chicken breast with green beans and asparagus	
10:30 pm	2 big bowls of cereal	Craving carbs – didn't have any for lunch or dinner.
Fri 7:30 am	Starbucks breakfast sandwich	Ran out of protein bars.
10:30 am	Yogurt and granola	
12:30 pm	Sandwich from work cafeteria	Ran out of salad stuff.
4:00 pm	Two handfuls granola	
7:00 pm	Fish filet with steamed broccoli and cauliflower	

TIME	FOOD	NOTES
9:00 p.m.	Entire sleeve of soda crackers	Trying to watch my carbs at night but then find myself obsessing about them for hours.
Sat 9:00 am	Omelet with bacon and cheddar, potatoes, toast, ½ cinnamon roll	Breakfast with Suzanne.
1:00 pm	Green salad with 1 can tuna	
6:00 pm	Vodka soda	Happy hour with Diane and Jim.
7:30 pm	Vodka martini, chips and salsa and guacamole, shared rolled tacos, cheese enchiladas, rice, beans, churros	Dinner with friends. Felt stuffed.
9:30 pm	3 vodkas with cranberry juice	Drinks with friends.
12:00 am	French fries and 2 slices of apple pie	Drunk- late night snacking. Craved comfort food not salad!
Sun 12:00 pm	4 egg whites, spinach and mushrooms	Trying not to eat too much to make up for last night ☹
3:15 pm	4 handfuls trail mix	Felt starving! Grabbed trail mix on impulse.
7:00 pm	Big salad with shrimp	Finally went to grocery store and food prepped a little for the week.

Although this is only one week of food logging, it might still be possible to identify some trends. I would definitely say one of Lauren's danger zones is social eating. It seems that when Lauren shares a meal with other people, her eating is over the top. It's also completely different from how she eats when she is alone.

Although it is not on our list, another danger zone that Lauren might have is grocery outage. Many people grocery shop once a week, but sometimes it needs to be more frequent than that. Lauren seemed to have a lot of healthy food choices available, but as her grocery supply diminished, she didn't step in and replenish it. As a result, her eating wasn't as varied and healthy as she would have liked.

Another danger zone that surfaces in this log relates to restricting carbohydrates to such a degree that Lauren struggled with cravings for bread, cereal, crackers, and the like. Getting overly hungry is another danger zone that made an appearance in Lauren's food log. If we had another week or two of logs, we would easily be able to see if these danger zones are a legitimate concern for Lauren and whether there are any others that can be addressed in this program.

Just to make sure you've fully understand how to use this food log, let's look at another example. This time it's Tracey's turn to unearth some Danger Zones.

TIME	FOOD	NOTES
Mon 6:30 am	2 hard-boiled eggs	Before workout.
8:30 am	Protein shake	After workout.
3:00 pm	2 KitKat bars	Worked through lunch. Found these in the breakroom.
7:00 pm	Handful of Triscuits	Just got home.
8:00 pm	Lasagna	Leftovers from last night.
Tues 6:30 am	2 hard-boiled eggs	Before workout.
8:30 am	Protein shake	After workout.
10:30 am	Bag of Cheetos	From breakroom.
3:15 pm	Ham sandwich	Worked through lunch. Someone brought sandwiches in.
6:45 pm	Handful of Triscuits	Just got home.
7:45 pm	Amy's frozen Dinner	
Weds 6:30 am	2 Hard –boiled eggs	Before workout.
8:30 am	Protein shake	After workout.
2:30 pm	Almonds, chocolate, chips	Grabbed from breakroom on my way to meeting.
4:30 pm	Almonds, chocolate, chips	Grabbed after my meeting.
7:30 pm	Lots of Triscuits	Just got home and was starving.
8:00 pm	Amy's frozen dinner	
Thurs 7:30 am	Muffin	No workout- got muffin from work.
9:45 am	Banana	
12:30 pm	Salad	From the restaurant across the street.

TIME	FOOD	NOTES
3:30 pm	Almonds	From the breakroom.
7:15 pm	Handful Triscuits	Just got home.
7:45 pm	Frozen pizza	
Fri 6:30 am	2 hard-boiled eggs	Before workou.t
08:30 am	Protein shake	After workout.
10:45 am	Cottage cheese	Brought from home.
2:30 pm	Almonds and chocolate	Running to a meeting again.
4:30 pm	2 slices pizza	In the breakroom.
8:00 pm	Mahi Mahi with green beans and mashed potatoes 1 roll, 1 glass wine	Dinner out.
Sat 7:45 am	Scrambled eggs with mushrooms and onions, 1 piece toast	
11:00 am	Triscuits	
1:30 pm	Subway 6-inch turkey sandwich	
6:30 pm	Amy's frozen dinner	
8:30 pm	Popcorn	Movies with a friend.
Sun 9:30 am	Omelet- cheese and avocado, fruit, toast	Breakfast with friend.
12:00 pm	Handful of Triscuits	
2:30 pm	Quesadilla	
6:45 pm	Frozen pizza	

Tracey's food log is certainly different from Lauren's. For Tracey, most of her danger zones are work-related. For example, it looks like both Tracey's breakroom at work and the transition between work and home are danger zones for her. It's also possible that some of the eating Tracey does at work is because work stress is also a danger zone for her.

When you look at Tracey's food log in detail, it shows that she often works through lunch and then over-snacks later in the day—usually on whatever she can find in the breakroom. Tracey also seems to "celebrate" her return home with a handful of Triscuits, regardless of whether she is hungry. It's a habitual response that Tracey might not have even noticed, had it not been for this food-log exercise. Unlike Lauren, it doesn't look like Tracey's eating becomes extreme when she goes out to restaurants or attends social situations.

Are you starting to get a feel for this? Now, it's time to look at your own eating by filling in food logs during the next couple of weeks. Remember, just write down what you are eating, when you eat it, and any relevant comments. Do not worry about changing what, when, and how much you are eating. This is simply a data-collecting process. It is meant to help pave the way for you to create action plans that will effectively address your particular danger zones.

Remember, we are just looking for trends—when does your eating deviate from the norm? When does your eating appear to be least controlled? When does your eating feel problematic? If you are not sure, then a couple of weeks of food logs should help you answer those questions. If you are still unsure, e-mail me your food logs, and I'll let you know what I think!

As for those of you who are *well aware* of your danger zones, well, you've already won half the battle. Knowing your problem areas makes it that much easier to solve them—and that's exactly what the next chapter is all about.

MY FOOD LOG, WEEK ONE		
TIME	FOOD	NOTES

MY FOOD LOG, WEEK ONE		
TIME	**FOOD**	**NOTES**

MY FOOD LOG, WEEK ONE		
TIME	**FOOD**	**NOTES**

MY FOOD LOG, WEEK TWO		
TIME	FOOD	NOTES

MY FOOD LOG, WEEK TWO		
TIME	**FOOD**	**NOTES**

MY FOOD LOG, WEEK TWO		
TIME	**FOOD**	**NOTES**

CHAPTER 16

Actions Plans: Taking the Danger Out of Danger Zones

"We delight in the beauty of the butterfly, but rarely admit the changes it has gone through to achieve that beauty."

—MAYA ANGELOU

Hopefully, at this point you are clear about your danger zones. That might be because you were already aware of them before delving into the last chapter. Or maybe, it's because you've done a few weeks of food logging, which helped you identify the danger zones that are worth addressing. Either way, it is now time to create action plans to counteract those danger zones.

Counteracting danger zones can mean many different things. It can mean avoiding danger zones altogether. (I mean, when is there ever a real need to let yourself get overly hungry?) It can also mean developing healthy coping skills you can use when you encounter a danger zone (so that it eventually becomes a not-so-dangerous zone). And it can mean planning an early escape from a situation that is making it hard for you to eat in a way that feels calm, relaxed, and healthy.

Earlier I talked about my difficulty with business trips. Those were the trips that would see me stand by as all my healthy habits disappeared into thin air. Once I understood this type of traveling to be my danger zone, I could put together my own action plan. As soon as I did that, my experience of going away for business completely changed (thank goodness, for that)! Here is a summary of the action plan I put together to address the danger zone that had developed around my work travel.

Action Item 1—
Commit to Exercising Each Day of My Trip

I made this commitment with the understanding that it didn't have to be the most intense, hardcore workout imaginable—it just had to be exercise. And, for the record, exercise for me includes walking through a local neighborhood, doing yoga while watching the six o'clock news, or making use of the hotel gym. There were all sorts of options that I could choose from. So, if all I could fit in was 15 minutes—then all I did 15 minutes. The point was just to do it. Why did I include exercise in my action plan? Exercising always makes me feel better, healthier, and leaves me much less likely to use food to meet emotional needs.

Action Item 2—
Always Take What I Call "Travel Food" on My Trips

For me, this is usually a handful of protein bars, some nuts, individual packets of nut butters, and Larabars (made with fruits and nuts), and roasted chick pea snacks. These foods travel well and cover me for snacking, ensuring that I don't get overly hungry and tempted. When I'm in a strange city and I need a snack, I can go to the hotel gift shop and get a bag of chips, but I can also choose to eat a handful of walnuts or a Larabar. Having my travel food with me ensures that I don't eat junk food out of desperation. (I'm all for having a bag of chips when I want one, but I'm not into eating a bag of chips because I haven't planned ahead and don't have many other options.)

Action Item 3—
Allow for One Indulgence a Day

I love food, and eating at new places is one of my favorite things about traveling, but I was going way overboard. If I wanted to have an indulgent breakfast, I could do that. But as much as I like to indulge, I also like feeling healthy. So, in keeping with the 80/20 approach, an indulgent breakfast would be followed by a lighter, more nutritious lunch and dinner. (And by lighter, I don't mean "diet," I just mean foods that don't feel quite so heavy.) This was a good compromise for me, as it allowed me to experience some food-related fun when I traveled, without finding myself feeling weighed down and bloated after an entire day of rich foods.

And guess what? My action plan worked. I was able to stick with it, because I felt accountable (after all I was the one who made it!) and because it was a balanced plan that didn't require long workouts or extreme food restriction. The result was, and still is, great. When I first started using this action plan, I took a written copy with me on my business trips. But after a while (maybe even 66 days?), I just got it, and now I don't even have to think about it. I just know that this is what I do when I travel.

Now, it's time to put together your action plans. Each plan should be specific for a particular danger zone and how your eating behavior changes when you encounter that situation. One thing to keep in mind is that danger zones usually involve mindless eating, or eating that is disconnected or numb. If you are familiar with mindful-eating techniques, you might want to consider including them in your action plan. If not, and you'd like to learn more, my full online Shatter the Yoyo program teaches mindful-eating techniques in-depth.

To help you get started on your action plans, I'll review some ideas that might help manage the danger zones we discussed previously. The list of ideas I am providing is not exhaustive so, by all means, add your own ideas to your personalized action plans. Feel free to take the ideas, play with them, and make them your own. Remember that creating an effective action plan might require testing a version, tweaking it here and there, and finally arriving at a final product that will consistently work for you.

Think of this process like an experiment! The most important thing is that you make it reasonable and easy to follow. If you don't, you run the risk of simply saying, "Screw it!" when the time comes to use your action plan. Had I made an action item that said, "No restaurant eating on business trips. Ever!" there's no way I would have been able to stick with it! It is so unrealistic that I would have quickly dropped the idea of doing anything to address the out-of-control eating that surfaced when I traveled for work. That is why you need to make your action items reasonable!

Restaurant Eating

Restaurant eaters tend to overindulge when they eat out—this is an extension of all-or-nothing thinking: I eat perfectly at home, so I can blow it all at a restaurant. Knowing this, action items should focus on limiting indulgences (experience it without *over*-experiencing it), allowing for eating out on a regular basis (so it doesn't feel scarce and like it needs to be taken advantage of), preparing for restaurant eating ahead of time (so you are not making decisions out of hunger—we make our worst decisions when we are hungry!), and allowing for occasional indulgences at home (so eating out isn't the only time you get to eat something special).

Action Item Examples

- Identify one special food/drink that would make the meal. It could be a drink, an appetizer, or a dessert. If you're contemplating ordering all three, ask yourself if all-or-nothing thinking is having an impact.

- If you can make it work with your schedule and finances, make restaurant eating a regular event. You won't feel the need to "grab while the getting is good," if you know you'll be going out again shortly.

- Ask the waiter to serve you half the entrée and wrap the other half to go. (Of course, if you're hungry enough to eat the whole meal, then go for it. But if you know that you'll eat everything on your plate purely out of habit, then this might be a good action item for you.)

- Allow special treats or indulgences at home several times a week

- Review menus and decide what to eat ahead of time. This might help if you're the type who gets overwhelmed by a menu chock-full of enticing options.

- If you are really hungry, have a snack before going to dinner, so you don't overindulge purely because you waited too long between meals.

Social Events

If food and social activities combine to equal overindulgence for you, then an action plan will help you appreciate the event without leaving feeling overly full and guilty. Action items for this danger zone should focus on preplanning, using the 80/20 approach to your advantage, and practicing behavior that will help break old, unhealthy patterns.

Action Item Examples

- Look at all the food options. Choose one item that stands out above the rest and enjoy it thoroughly. If you're going to go for multiple special foods, make sure it is out of hunger and not a reaction to all the dieting you've done throughout the years.

- Sitting while you're eating makes it much harder to get swept up in mindless eating.

- If you are likely to feel like a kid in a candy store, who wants everything she/he sees, consider deciding what you will eat ahead of time. Of course, that's not always possible. When it is, deciding beforehand can make room in your head for the social part of the evening, rather than letting questions about what you are going to eat take up all the room.

- Have a snack before the event, so that extreme hunger doesn't drive extreme eating.

- Settle in somewhere other than next to the food table. This is another way of making sure that mindless eating doesn't make an appearance during the social gathering.

- Think carefully before you go for a second round at the buffet table. If you're physically hungry, then it's a go. But if you're eating because your mind, rather than your body, is hungry, look for something else to do. Talk to a friend, help clean up, or step outside for a breath of fresh air.

- Limit your alcoholic drinks—decide beforehand how many you'll have. If you go overboard with drinking, mindless eating is often not far behind.

- Have a glass of water between alcoholic drinks. That can keep you from mindlessly drinking too much.

- If you're not hungry when you arrive, postpone eating until you're hungry enough to truly enjoy the food. (Just don't postpone eating until you're starving. That's just inviting a different danger zone to the party!)

- Consider ending your eating two hours after arriving. Not as an arbitrary, diet-related rule, but to help make sure that mindless grazing through the food tables isn't how you spend the evening.

Business Meals

The business meal danger zone is about going to restaurants or ordering in as part of a work meeting. Hopefully, you'll reach a point where you are confident enough about your own eating plan that you won't give a second thought to the (unsolicited) opinions of others. However, when business meetings are a danger zone, the problem is often related to image (for example, "What will people think if I only order a salad and they all have steak?") or lack of control related to restaurant eating. If it is more related to the general restaurant eating danger zone, review some of the action items under that heading. When the business meal danger zone is you worrying about what others will think about your menu choices, action items should focus on preplanning and self-talk.

Action Item Examples

- Decide what you are going to eat/order ahead of time, so you don't let the judgment of others steer you in the wrong direction.

- Try to be the first to order. Your colleagues might still comment, but at least you won't be tempted to change your selection, based on the orders that went before you.

- If it is truly necessary to be left in peace by your colleagues, mention that you are not hungry before ordering. Eventually, using this program, you'll learn not to feel the need to excuse or explain what, when, and how much you eat.

- Write a list of reasons why what you are ordering has no impact on the meeting. Read it to yourself before going to the business meal.

- Come up with a witty, polite, and professional comeback, if one of the other attendees starts to question your food choices. For example, "Thanks for the suggestion, Bill. But what I ordered is exactly what I need to keep my focus on tonight's business. If I fill up on rich food tonight, I won't be able to do my share of the work and that wouldn't be fair to anyone."

Being Home Alone

If your danger zone is being home alone, you are likely prone to hiding your eating from others. You might think that being alone is your only opportunity to eat certain off-limits foods. This can leave you feeling compelled to binge when no one is around. If that's the case, then you need to focus on either keeping yourself busy, keeping yourself with others, and/or addressing the drive to overeat in privacy.

Action Item Examples

- Determine when you are most likely to be alone at home and make plans—invite a friend over, go to a gym class, go for a walk, go to the movies, etc.

- Ensure that you remove the stigma from previously off-limits foods. Allowing yourself to eat them on a "normal" day, reduces the risk that you'll binge on them when home alone.

- If you are home alone and feeling the urge to binge, have a list of activities that you can use to distract yourself. Here are some ideas: Put in a load of laundry, read Facebook for 15 minutes, do 5 minutes of ab exercises, make some hot tea, or read a book. Make sure the distractions are enjoyable or satisfying in some way. If you don't, the activities might not be sufficiently interesting to keep you out of the cupboards and fridge.

- Create a list of rewards you can chose from each time you successfully avoid bingeing when home alone. It might be a pedicure, a new lipstick, a trip to the movies, or something else that celebrates this achievement.

Food "Pushers" and/or Family Pressure

Food pushers create a unique danger zone, because you're not the manager of their behavior, you're just at the receiving end. But, you can be the manager of how you respond to the food pushers' never-ending desire to have you eat some more. Usually, you're likely to know exactly where, and when, your food pushers will be most active. Perhaps, it's anytime you go over to their house. Or, maybe it's at family events. Whatever the case might be, knowing when you are risk of being cornered by a food pusher allows you to prepare in advance. Being prepared means that instead of having a piece of Aunt Gladys' (overly sweet) pecan pie, you have other options.

Action Item Examples

- Try to be the cook in any situation involving your food pushers. It's hard for even the most blatant food pusher to try to get you to eat more of your own food!
- If they need to bring something, suggest they bring something that is unlikely to cause conflict. Food pushers aren't known for trying to get people to eat a second bowl of garden salad.
- Prepare a short, unemotional, yet respectful response (for example, "No, thank you. I just ate," or "That looks great, maybe I'll have it later"). Don't overexplain. That just gives the food pushers more opportunity to argue back.
- Try to schedule experiences with food pushers that do not revolve around food (for example, go for a walk, see a movie, go to an art gallery, or go shopping).

Boredom

If boredom is a frequent danger zone for you, it's time to address why you're bored. As entirely eliminating boredom isn't likely, it's also important to have a list of positive (or, at the least, neutral) activities that you can turn to when bored.

Action Item Examples

- Take a look at your food logs. Is there a time of the day and/or week when you're most likely to engage in boredom eating? If so, make a plan specifically for those times. If it's Sunday night at 6 p.m. when boredom and the urge to eat come-a-knocking, then why not make that the night that you (a) go to yoga class, (b) finally start reading that great novel that has essentially set up roots on your bedside table, or (c) catch up with your best friend over a cup of herbal tea?

- If you're about to, or have already begun to, boredom eat, call a time out. Spend the next 60 seconds doing some type of physical activity. It could be jumping jacks or could be dancing to this week's top 40 songs. The point is, exercise can "perk" you up enough that your boredom won't lead you to the kitchen so readily.

- Just as for the being home alone action plan, boredom eating is less likely if you have a list of things to do as an alternative to finishing off a box of cookies. Make sure that this list is ready and waiting, because boredom eating doesn't always give you a lot of notice. Activities that my clients have used to get through this danger zone include calling a friend, working on a jigsaw puzzle, going for a walk, reading, (finally!) organizing their closets, and crafts, like knitting and sewing.

- Speaking of crafts, if you find yourself bored a lot, it makes sense to try out a new hobby. But if this hobby is going to offer any protection against boredom eating, make sure it is something you can do without much preparation and most anywhere. So, drawing in a sketchbook would fit the bill. Recreational sailing, while offering all sorts of benefits, is not the most convenient antidote to boredom eating!

TV Watching/Snacking

For those of you who struggle with snacking during TV watching, the focus is on breaking the association between food and the screen. Instead, create a new habit. You can learn to associate the television with that 15 minutes of stretching that your healthcare professional told you to do three times a week. Or maybe watching television is the perfect time to fold all that laundry that is ready and waiting in the dryer. The point is, if you can eat and watch television, you can do something healthy while watching television. Find what works the best for you and prepare to give up snacking for a habit that will leave you healthier and happier.

While you're waiting to find the new (and better) habit, you can also deliberately break the patterns associated with eating in front of the television. So, if it's your tradition to have pizza night in front of the tube every Friday, but the pizza night quickly becomes the pizza and ice cream and chips and way-too-many-cookies night, then plan to eat the pizza at the table, put the leftovers away (every single crumb!) and only then, watch television.

Action Item Example

- Sit in a spot you don't usually sit in to watch TV.
- Use a stress ball or grip strengthener to keep your hands active while watching TV.
- Create a kitchen closure time—a time after which you no longer spend time in the kitchen, unless you are truly, without-a-doubt, physically hungry. If you find yourself in the kitchen for any other reason, an urge to screen eat might be the reason why.
- If you feel a craving to get a snack while watching TV, do something else—exercise, dance, knit, crossword puzzles, etc.
- If you haven't yet been able to break the connection between the screen and excessive snacking, consider reducing the amount of time you spend in front of the

television. Once you are more confident that you won't fall back into bad habits while watching your favorite program, you can up your TV watching. In the meantime, consider doing something else instead of plopping yourself down in front the screen. You can write, read, walk, play with your pets, etc.

Transitioning from Work to Home

If your danger zone is in the adjustment from work to home, there are two things that might be going on. One is that you simply are hungry—for most people it is almost dinner time, after all! (If you're a shift worker and find yourself coming home in the morning, a change to your sleep cycle might also be contributing to a tendency to overeat.) The second is that snacking has become the ritual you use to announce the end of the work day and the start of the "home" day.

Action Item Examples

- If it's excessive hunger that has you munching frantically when you get home, eat a snack right before leaving work or while heading home.

- Go for a walk as soon as you get home—this can become your new, healthy ritual.

- Or, for the same reason, do five minutes of exercise right when you get home.

- If it's "a break" you're looking for after a long day at work, find a place (other than the kitchen) where you can read the newspaper, leaf through a magazine, or watch the news. Do anything that feels like a "break" but doesn't involve mindlessly eating 16 crackers, three cookies, and a big handful of trail mix.

- If those options don't work for you, experiment with other rituals you can do after returning home. A 15-minute power nap, a quick shower, a snuggle with your dog/cat/ guinea pig, or one of those adult coloring books are other possible rituals.

Work Stress

If work stress is causing you to turn to food, the quickest solution is to find something other than eating that can give you a break from the pressure you're feeling. The longer-term solution is to step back from your work and consider whether there is anything you can do to reduce the amount of stress that it generates.

Action Item Examples

- Take a walk around the building every hour.
- Close your door and meditate for five minutes. (There are all sorts of apps that can guide you through a short meditation.)
- Take a Facebook break every hour to clear your head. (Just make sure your workplace is Facebook friendly!)
- Anytime you feel yourself turning to food, do one minute of squats or push-ups instead. If those exercises are too vigorous, stretching is another great alternative. Try a few neck and back stretches at your desk.
- Lie down on the floor in your office and breathe deeply for a couple of minutes.
- Play a game on your phone or computer (if allowed). Solitaire, anyone?
- Go outside for a fresh air break.
- Take five minutes to debrief with a supportive colleague.

- Longer term, think of ways to organize your work life that reduce the routine stress associated with your job. Remember chronic stress is not your appetite's friend!

Traveling

If traveling is your danger zone (as it is mine!), then your action plan will involve changing your mindset. When it is a danger zone, traveling becomes an opportunity to open the floodgates and eat everything in sight. It is that outlook that needs to be reset. Creating a "travel plan" can be quite helpful.

Action Item Examples

- Pick one meal each day that will be more indulgent than others. That should help you achieve the 80/20 balance when it comes to your healthy eating/indulgent eating split.
- Take travel snack food with you to avoid becoming overly hungry or having no choice but to eat foods that historically have triggered bingeing (for example, chocolate bars, chips, doughnuts).
- Plan pleasurable activities in your travel day so you have something to look forward to other than food.
- Focus on including vegetables in every meal and snack on fruits. Both foods can help combat the sluggish feeling that traveling can often bring and which can encourage "fatigue" eating.
- Pick one meal each day that is going to be clean/real food. Just like fruits and vegetables, this can help give you the energy and motivation you need to make healthy, life-affirming food choices.

Buffets/Parties

As mentioned earlier, this mentality is often about taking advantage of freebies. An important question to ask yourself is, "Why do I need to take advantage of it?" Follow that with a second question, "Is the outcome, (feeling crappy, gaining weight, feeling bad about myself) worth saving a few bucks?"

Action Item Examples

- Take a lap through the whole buffet before plating. Once you know all the choices, decide which foods you would truly enjoy.

- Predetermine the amount of times you are going to get a refill at the buffet. It's important to not let this be an in-the-moment decision, driven by old habits.

- Start with salad or vegetables in your first course. This isn't meant as the old diet standby of filling up on low-calorie foods so you don't have room for dessert. Rather, this is meant to ensure that you don't lose sight of your health, just because you're in a room full of free (or close to it), formerly off-limits foods.

- Order time-consuming items in your second course (for example, omelet station). That can give you the time to reflect, pause, and determine if you're truly hungry (or whether you're now eating because you just can't resist a freebie).

- Ask yourself, "If it wasn't free, would I eat it/buy it?" If the answer is, "No," then don't.

- Eat before going to the party, if you're hungry. The last thing you want do is compound the "freebie" danger zone with being overly hungry.

Snacking at Work

If this is your danger zone, an action plan is almost always about limiting your access to food that you're likely to eat "just because" rather than due to physical hunger. Finding alternatives to mindless eating and setting up barriers to the easy access can form the basis of some of your action items.

Action Item Examples

- Have a "no freebies" policy. If you want it, go to the store, and get it for yourself. This prevents the freebie danger zone from triggering a snacking at work danger zone.

- Create your own snack drawer filled with foods that you like and which support your health. This gives you a choice between eating the breakroom potato chips that you don't even like and the healthy Larabar that really hits the spot when you're hungry.

- Find alternative walking routes, so you don't have to pass by the breakroom so frequently. Out of sight, out of mind comes in handy in this case.

- Create an "exercise before snacking rule." For example, do one minute of squats or push-ups before getting anything from the breakroom. Exercise can release feel-good chemicals in your brain, helping to prevent the stress-eating danger zone that can surface at work.

Too Tired, Lazy, Stressed to Cook

If you find that laziness about cooking is often your danger zone, then you need to parcel out time to cook during those times that you actually are motivated to do so. To really make your action plan effective, try not to make just one meal when you're cooking. Use your time in the kitchen to double or triple up. That way, you'll end up with multiple meals you can use when you're just too darn tired to start cutting up vegetables.

Action Item Examples

- Plan a food prep hour on Sunday nights (or any night that works in your schedule). Make things that will be quick and easy to reheat (casseroles, chicken dishes, stir fry, etc.) when you need them later in the week.
- When you cook anything, make a double or triple batch and freeze the extras. Next time you're hungry and tired, all you need to do is a quick microwave heat-up!
- Stock up with healthy, quick meals—(canned soups, tuna fish pouches, canned beans, veggie burgers, etc.)
- Have a "no delivery" rule. If you order out, you're going to go get it! That will make you pause long enough to determine if you're entering an order out danger zone or whether you're making a reasonable choice to have pizza for dinner.

Junk Food around the House

This danger zone almost always relates to others in the house—usually significant others or children. It can also relate to baking supplies, if you're someone who likes to whip up a batch of chocolate chip cookies for the office from time to time. The action items usually relate to limiting your access and any visual cues.

Action Item Examples

- Ask your significant other to limit the junk he or she brings into the house. If they feel a need to bring in a quart of mint chocolate chip ice cream (your favorite, no less!), ask them to hide it somewhere out of sight. After all, the back of the freezer is just as good a place for ice cream as the front.

- Have a kid's snack cabinet that is separate from your pantry. Now you don't have to see, and be tempted by, their snacks multiple times a day.
- Consider replacing your kids' junk food with healthier options that they still enjoy but which don't leave you at risk of danger zone eating.
- Utilize a storage area outside the kitchen for junk food. In my experience, the garage is a great option.
- Throw out special occasion food when the occasion is over (birthday cake is for the birthday)!
- If you're a baker and want to have chocolate chips, marshmallows, and pralines on hand, store them in a nontransparent tote that you can put out of sight. Maybe that means the garage again—or the back of the top cupboard, a spot you can't reach without getting the stepladder out. This will reduce the risk that you'll grab a handful of chocolate chips just because they are within arm's reach.

Sensory Cravers

If you are a sensory craver, then your action items need to focus on ways to limit your exposure to sensory overload situations. Also, find healthy ways to respond once your senses trigger an urge to eat and eat and eat.

Action Item Examples

- Keep emergency snack food on your person when you are out (especially at the mall)! This way the smell of

Cinnabon, Mrs. Fields Cookies, and KFC don't have to lead you astray.

- Exercise during television commercials to remove your focus from the sight of food, and shift it to how good it feels to move, stretch, and get your blood flowing.

- Skip television commercials by watching prerecorded shows or Netflix.

- Eat before you go shopping. Being overly hungry will heighten your sensations and put you at risk of buying a box of Twinkies simply because they look so yummy.

Late-Night Snacking

If you are a late-night snacker, chances are that you are doing this out of habit more than anything else. Now is the time to create new bedtime habits that can replace much of your end-of-day snacking.

Action Item Examples

- Create a kitchen closure time—a time at which you can no longer go into the kitchen. You can flex, if you're truly hungry, but otherwise, stay away when you know you've had enough to eat for the night.

- Create a soothing bedtime ritual—tea, eye mask, meditation, reading, bath, etc. This can help distract you from the snacking habit that you've ritualized throughout the years.

- Journal instead of giving in to cravings. Write about your cravings and how you are feeling. You might discover that what you really need is a hug, to talk to a friend, or to go to bed and catch up on your sleep.

- Drink water if having a full stomach makes it easier to fall asleep.

Reward Eating ("I Deserve a Treat.")

If reward eating is your danger zone, now is the time to come up with a long list of others way to recognize a job well done, a mission accomplished, or a special event (such as your birthday or a work promotion).

Action Item Examples

- Make a list of small, but special, things that bring joy to your life. A bubble bath perhaps? A new nail polish? A favorite magazine? A foot massage from your spouse? The next time you deserve a reward, work your way through this list instead of working your way through the kitchen.
- Using food to reward yourself doesn't have to result in out of control, danger-zone type eating. Just make sure you choose a special food and eat it when you're truly hunger. Don't just overeat anything that happens to be handy as a reward—because in the longer term that kind of eating is not a reward, it's more like a punishment.

"I'm So Tired!" Eating

If you tend to overeat when you're tired, then the absolute best solution is to add more sleep to your daily schedule. If you're rolling your eyes because you're a new mom, work shifts, or have struggled with insomnia for the past 10 years, it might help to know that even if you can't sleep more, you can learn to navigate this danger zone without relying so much on food.

Action Item Examples

- If you haven't done this already, find ways to improve your sleep circumstances. This might mean making your room darker, turning off your screens earlier in the evening, or buying yourself the best pillow ever.

- If circumstances beyond your control are interfering with your sleep, find ways to support yourself through the day that don't include eating bowls of leftover pasta just to get through the day. Take a cool shower, stretch while the baby is settled for a bit, ask your partner to make dinner so you can take a power nap, or invest in a babysitter who can be your eyes and ears while you snooze for a few hours.

- Take an honest look at your schedule and identify the things that really can be delayed or dropped entirely. Some people are so busy meeting other people's needs that they don't leave themselves enough sleeping time. If you really need a nap, then maybe now's not the time to help your friend organize her garage.

 **Take Action:** Now it's your turn to put together your own action plans. Go through the list and suggestions in this chapter. You can use the examples provided to make your action plans or make something entirely new based on your needs and preferences. Once you come up with your most important action plans (as determined by your most challenging danger zones), write them on the "My Danger Zone Action Plan" provided at the end of this chapter.

Next, start the implementation phase. Don't wait until you have the perfect-sure-to-be-100 percent-effective action plan!

Remember, action plans usually involve some trial and error—you'll have to try your action plans, and then tweak them to find what works the best. That is absolutely okay!

Above all, remember that this takes practice! Your old ways of reacting to danger zones are long-standing habits, so don't expect them to change overnight. You might have to practice your action plans for months before they become second nature, but it will be time and effort well spent. If you stop practicing before your action plans become automatic, danger zones might continue to derail your weight management goals for the foreseeable future.

My Danger Zone Action Plan

Danger Zone: _____

Action Plan

1. _____
2. _____
3. _____
4. _____
5. _____

Danger Zone: _____

Action Plan

1. _____
2. _____
3. _____
4. _____
5. _____

Danger Zone: _____

Action Plan

1. _____
2. _____
3. _____
4. _____
5. _____

Stacking the Odds in Your Favor

CHAPTER 17
The Power of Self-Care

*"Love yourself first and everything else falls in line.
You really have to love yourself to get anything done in
this world."*

—LUCILLE BALL

When we talk about food restriction, it is also important to talk about self-care. At first glance, if might seem like those two concepts don't go together. But, let's take a closer look. We have talked about how restriction leads to bingeing, an extreme version of emotional eating, which is compounded by the mind and body's biological reaction to restricting calories. I focus much more in-depth on emotional eating and mindfulness in my full Shatter the Yoyo program, but here I want to talk a little bit about combatting emotional eating.

By removing restrictions, you can begin the process of ending the control food has over you. And by putting an end to that control, you are taking an important step toward putting an end to binge eating. However, that also means putting an end to eating vast amounts of food for comfort. This means that your need for comfort will have to be met in a different way. That's where self-care comes into play.

Self-care comes in a variety of shapes and sizes. For some people, it means making sure they check their blood sugar regularly. For others, it means setting aside or "protecting" time for themselves, so that the day isn't a haze of work, chores, and doing favors. Self-care means being able to say "no" when you need a break more than anything and someone wants you to write one more report, work one more shift, or host one more dinner.

Most people are busy, busy, busy nowadays. With that kind of go-go-go lifestyle, it can be easy to let things slip. And often it is the things that you do for yourself that are the first to suffer. This program requires commitment and energy, and you might find both of these in short supply if you don't recharge and rejuvenate yourselves from time to time. As the old saying goes, all work and no play, makes Jane (John) a dull (and tired!) woman (man).

Another important factor to look at is the nature of how you take care of yourself. How you take care of yourself and prioritize your health is a direct representation of how you see yourself and how you present yourself to the world. What does it say about you if your health and wellness is only a priority *temporarily?* Your health and wellness should always be a priority. That is exactly why creating a healthy lifestyle has so much more value than simply going on a diet.

Self-care should be customized to your life and your needs, wants, and habits. As an example, there are quite a few people who really need to cut down on the amount of screen time they have in their life. Hours spent on the phone and/or computer come at a cost, which can directly and indirectly make weight loss that much harder.

For most of us, a good majority of our day is spent in front of a screen. We wake up, check our phone, read Facebook, watch the news as we get ready for our day, sit in front of a computer all day at work, come home and watch TV, and go to bed with our phones. We wake up the next morning, and the cycle starts all over again!

When it comes to weight and health, the most significant screen time, and the time we are going to focus on, is the end-of-the-day/after-work screen time. Let's look at those after-work hours of your day when you are engaging in screen time. If you watch television, what else are you doing during this time? The most common answers to that question are (1) sitting, and (2) snacking. Can you see why this might be a problem? The complete and total inactivity that comes with evening screen time is a huge part of the issue.

Joining inactivity as a problem is the fact that being on screen is often coupled with mindless snacking. (And let's not even get into all the messages about eating you get from television commercials!) So, the more evening screen time you have, the less active you are, the more your metabolism shuts off, and, at the same time, you are filling up with snack food that is often not particularly healthy. Not a great formula for weight management, right? This is backed by massive amounts of research showing a connection between television viewing time and obesity!

 **Take Action:** The bottom line is that most people need to fix this pattern by limiting their screen time. And here's the approach that I suggest: Figure out how much time you spend on a screen for personal reasons during the course of a day. Include time spent on your phone, tablet, laptop, desktop, or television—it all counts. If your screen time varies from day to day, then track it during a few days and calculate the average.

Now, here's the important part, cut that number in half. Yep, that's right, half. That is your goal for screen time! Let's say the

TV usually goes on at 7:00 p.m. and you watch until 10:00 p.m., and then you spend an hour on your phone in bed. That's a total of four hours of screen time. Your goal now is two hours. This means that you can have two hours of screen time in the evening, and the other two hours . . . well, they are going to have to be filled with something else! Maybe you take a walk, make a phone call, engage in a project, clean out a closet, read a book, play with your dog, meditate, do laundry—or maybe even a little bit of everything on that list. The actual mix of activities doesn't really matter—what matters is that you are doing something other than watching a screen. Sure, it might be a real shock to your system, but the more you practice "screen free" living, the easier it gets (and, in some cases, the better you'll sleep)! So, start practicing as soon as possible!

Screen time is a universal self-care issue but, in general, self-care for one person can look different from another person's version of self-care. What unites self-care in all its forms is that it involves giving yourself what you need to thrive, to feel both valued and valuable, and to optimize your health. The opposite is self-neglect.

Self-neglect can mean depriving yourself of things you love (a day of cocooning) or need (sleep) because you feel you aren't worth it or don't deserve it. Self-neglect can also mean not attending to you own health needs (ignoring troubling symptoms; forgetting to do the bloodwork your healthcare professional ordered; missing your morning blood pressure pill).

What does self-care include? Well, a lot of different activities can fall under that category but there are some common themes that come up again and again.

Environmental Self-Care

Sometimes, it can feel like your life is on hold until you conquer this whole weight thing. It consumes your thinking for much of the day and can leave little room for taking care of yourself in other ways. For example, you might put off creating a home or office environment that generates positive feelings. I mean, what's the point of having a beautiful home when you feel so ugly yourself, right? Well, have you ever had the experience of walking into a room, a store, or a business, and noticed your mood get a little brighter? You can thank any number of factors—natural light, warm colors, just-the-right amount of art, an impressively organized bookshelf . . . and on and on.

In contrast, environments that are cluttered, dirty, and crowded, can leave you feeling overwhelmed and without a single ounce of motivation to do anything. Ever. That's a doozy of an impact. And yet, despite there being a known association between our environment and our emotional health, it's not uncommon for people to tolerate clutter, to live out of boxes rather than finally(!) unpacking them, and to accept a disorganized (and frustrating) office as a permanent part of their life. You might ask, "So, now I need to clean my house and organize my work papers to lose weight!?" and the answer, of course, is, "No, you don't."

For one, some people claim that they thrive in mess, so if's that the case, mess away. For two, remember this program—the ain't-nobody-looking for perfection program? Well, that applies here too. You don't have to work miracles or change lifelong habits, but you do need to realize that you might be making your weight-loss efforts a lot harder by living in your own version of chaos. If you know in your heart of hearts that living in a cluttered, messy house is depleting you, then yes, self-care does mean doing some work on your environment. Even 15 minutes of effort can be a step toward creating a home that makes you smile rather than mindlessly eat. What are some of the things you can do to provide a "self-caring" environment? Well, try these on for size.

> Make your bed—fluff the pillows, smooth the blankets. Small things can make a big difference to how you feel when you come home after a long day.

> Finally put up the poster you got at the art show six months ago. It can brighten your room and your mood.

> Organize the shelf that now holds a pile of books and magazines and a random assortment of trinkets (and is about to topple).

> Create a relaxation corner—maybe a favorite pillow, a yoga mat, a soft blanket, some candles, and a framed picture of your favorite landscape. Or maybe try something entirely different. The point is to create your own personal retreat that you can visit when you need a break from the hustle and bustle (and clutter)!

Biological Self-Care

Back to this again? Yep, sleep, hydration, delicious food that nourish your bodies, regular mealtime, and physical activity can all be part of a biological self-care plan. For example, there are many studies showing that irregular eating patterns (yep, there's that pesky skipped lunch again) are associated with higher body weights. Knowing that something is good for us apparently isn't enough, because enough sleep, regular meals, and (nonpunishing) exercise are all things that people often go without for extended periods of times. (Years, anyone?) Maybe because they haven't fully embraced the idea that they deserve to have a happy and healthy life. And, just to be clear, you deserve to have it now, not once you lose 20 pounds, finish going to school, or the kids are out of the house. Want some ideas of where to start when it comes to biological self-care? Check out these options.

> Don't shortchange yourself when it comes to sleep. Scientists know a lot about what not getting enough sleep can do to the human body (and it isn't pretty) that it's starting to look like sleep deprivation is right up there with smoking.

> Don't skip breakfast, don't skip lunch, and don't skip dinner. Many people also need to throw in a snack (or three) to keep their blood sugar even and their bodies properly nourished.

> Don't make every meal a rushed, haphazard affair. Find the time to make your favorite soup from scratch or stroll through your local farmers market, looking for the reddest strawberries and freshest bread. Filling yourself up with "it'll do" foods is practical at times but should be considered a last resort.

> Oh, your aching back and sore knees. Now's the time to finally book that massage that you've been putting off until you lose 10 pounds. After all, what if self-care (like, say, a massage) can help give you the energy and motivation you need to see this program through to its successful end? Then all your waiting for "someday when I'm thin . . . " is actually what is keeping someday so far in the future.

Psychological Self-Care

The ins and outs of psychological needs could easily fill a book of their own. This is the short and sweet version. Everyone has certain preferences—maybe it's for alone time, maybe it's for a walk in the woods to clear the mind, or maybe it's not being subject to weight-related comments from Mom, Dad, or sis. Whatever it might be, these are all examples of the psychological self-care that can leave you feeling more resilient and less overwhelmed. Not everybody feels like they can speak up when their psychological needs aren't being met. Instead they grin and bear it (or eat and bear it). Developing the ability to be polite, but firm (assertive in other words), about your needs is an investment in your long-term health, including long-term weight management.

Why would psychological self-care translate to weight loss? For a whole bunch of reasons. It leaves you better able to manage stress without turning to food. By reducing stress, it keeps your hormones in check (the same hormones that can make your appetite go wild). The argument for psychological self-care has been so strong that a type of treatment called compassion-focused therapy (CFT) has been developed.

Studies on CFT have shown that being warm and compassionate toward yourself can improve mood, anxiety, and, yep, you guessed it, disordered eating, including binge eating. How great is that? Be nice to yourself, and your ability to have a healthy relationship with food gets better. That's reason enough to take psychological self-care seriously. Here are some other activities that fall under the same category.

> Block out the alone time you need to feel settled and calm. Maybe that means spending three hours at the library, leisurely browsing through the latest additions to the collection. Whatever alone time looks like for you, make time for those kinds of breaks.

> Create a list of power thoughts that leave you feeling hopeful, respected, and free of self-condemnation. Repeat them every day—more than once. Making time to give yourself this kind of pep talk will payoff.

➤ Set a boundary with friends or family who feel the need to sound off about your weight, your diet, or your life. Find a phrase that makes its point clearly and respectfully. Rehearse it out loud plenty of times. Then, close your eyes and imagine using it the next time a weight-based comment comes your way from dear Uncle Bob (or Aunt Shirley, or big sister Jackie, or boyfriend Mike). "I'm all for free speech, but I'm also all for treating people with kindness and respect. Your comments don't feel like either." Too strong? Not strong enough? Then come up with your own, so you don't have to dread the next family get together.

➤ Give mindfulness a shot. Many people report that this technique helps quiet all the judgmental "monkey chatter." Instead mindfulness is good chatter to quiet the judging of yourself, which can really undermine your efforts to be kind and tolerant toward yourself.

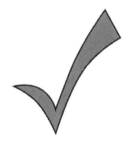

Take Action: Now it's your turn. Use the list in the Self-Care Worksheet to brainstorm something, anything, you can do to daily start taking care of your mind, body, and home. I've provided some examples, but like the rest of the program, you'll need to customize this tool to fit your life.

SELF-CARE WORKSHEET	
SELF- CARE: WHAT YOU NEED	SELF-CARE: HOW YOU'RE GOING TO DO IT
To eat lunch instead of skipping it because I'm "too busy."	Pack a favorite lunch the night before so it's ready to go to work with me the next day.
	As a reminder, set my watch alarm to go off 15 minutes before lunch.
	Make a lunch date with a friend – commit to not cancelling it!
Pretty up my kitchen so I enjoy coming home.	Buy a bouquet to brighten up the room.
	Set the timer for 15 minutes, and do a quick "clean and tidy". Any little progress counts.
	Invite a friend over for a "make my kitchen beautiful" consult.
Have a Saturday afternoon all to myself - time to recharge.	Rehearse a polite but firm statement you can use to decline requests and invitations.
	"Thank you for thinking of me but I have plans for the afternoon."
	"It sounds like a very worthy cause. Unfortunately, I'm so busy with my own project that I'm not able to help.

Now, your turn:

SELF-CARE: WHAT YOU NEED	SELF-CARE: HOW YOU'RE GOING TO DO IT

Case Study: When Rick Didn't Have Time for Rick

Rick was always in a hurry. Rushing in the morning to get to work on time, rushing to get his kids dropped off on time, and rushing to get them picked up while trying to beat traffic. As part of Rick's nonstop rushing during the workday, not eating enough for lunch was followed by eating too much at dinner and eating even more (usually ice cream) before bed. Rick truly believed he didn't have the time to do the hiking he loved. He also didn't have the time to go to bed before 11 (even though he was tired two hours earlier). Add to this the fact that Rick couldn't quite wrap his head around how much weight he had put on in the past few years, and something clearly wasn't working in Rick's life.

Rick had yoyo dieted as long as he could remember, but since the kids came, it seemed even harder to start a diet, let alone stick to it. Although he tried to push it to the back of his mind, Rick had a sneaking suspicion that no matter how hard he tried to resist, his weight was going to keep going up, up, and up. (And Rick was right. Not because he lacked willpower, smarts, or a desire to be thinner and healthier. But because his yoyo dieting habit was destined to keep his weight moving in the wrong direction).

When Rick first sought help for his weight, he was really looking for a diet coach. Someone who would teach him all the new tricks of the trade and help him stick to the straight and narrow once and for all. Instead, what he got with this program was encouragement to set aside time each day for self-care. Rick scoffed at the idea of self-care—did anyone have any idea how hard it was to balance being a father, a husband, and an employee? How was he supposed to magically come up with the time to do things for himself—taking away time from his other responsibilities wasn't possible. It would also be selfish according to Rick.

But perhaps there was another way of looking at it. Could Rick take a long hard look at his Facebook-at-night habit and maybe find a few more minutes of sleep? Could Rick and his wife give themselves permission to have a babysitter relieve them so they could go for a hike one Sunday afternoon a month? And maybe, just maybe, Rick would be even more productive at work, if he took the time to eat lunch, enjoy a walk around the block, and take a deep breath before getting back to his desk.

Rick was skeptical at first. His idea of using his time well was to be busy almost every minute of the day, except for his late-night screen and ice cream binges. But he could agree to changing his daily patterns for a couple of weeks—not because he truly believed self-care would work but because he considered himself a scientist and was willing to undertake an experiment.

Using the Shatter the Yoyo program worksheet, Rick identified a few self-activities he could introduce without shaking his current life to the core. He had to white knuckle through his not-so-much-time-in-front-of-screens evenings and felt a little panicky the first time he took an official lunch break at work. But, after two weeks, even Rick had to admit that he was feeling a little less overwhelmed, a little more energetic, and, yep, a little less hungry all the time. His work performance hadn't suffered, and his wife had noticed a difference in his mood at home.

It took Rick close to a year to slowly create a lifestyle that balanced his responsibilities and "to do" lists with the self-care he needed to fuel his weight-loss goals. It took a lot longer than a year for Rick to arrive at a weight that felt right for him. Rick's new approach to life (and eating) generally followed the 80/20 split. His ongoing goal was to put aside 20 percent of his nonwork/nonsleep time for self-care. His nutrition plan was also designed to work, even if 20 percent of the time his eating was less than ideal.

Rick persevered, despite the setbacks that happen anytime old habits are being changed. Rick's hard work and patience paid off, because this time when he hit his goal weight, he stayed there. Rick couldn't help but regret all those years he spent yoyo dieting when what he really needed to do was take the time to care for himself and stop dieting. If he had only known . . .

CHAPTER 18

Adding to Your "No More Yoyo Dieting" Toolbox

"Believe you can and you're halfway there."
—THEODORE ROOSEVELT

The core principles of this program include goal setting, challenging cognitive distortion, and adopting beliefs that provide support, as you make a clean break from yoyo dieting. These tools might be all that you need to reach your goal of successful, sustained weight management. Still, it is nice to know that there are even more skills that you can use to make reaching your goals easier and faster. We have Dr. Aaron Beck to thank for the cognitive behavioral skills discussed earlier.

Now, it's Dr. Marsha Linehan's turn. Dr. Linehan is a renowned psychologist who has done a lot of work helping people manage their distress in ways that don't make their lives even more difficult. Instead of coping with negative emotions by smoking, drinking, self-harming, or overeating, a person can turn to dialectical behavior therapy (DBT), the treatment developed by Dr. Linehan. DBT involves learning a whole host of skills that can help you create a "life worth living" rather than struggling with unhealthy habits, including emotional or binge eating. Different skills work for different people, but three DBT skills that I have seen benefit a lot of people are opposite action, wise mind, and distraction.

Opposite Action

Opposite action is a simple yet powerful skill. It helps you change the way you behave in response to cognitive distortions, including those that drive your on-again, off-again dieting. Of course, it would be great if you never had a distorted thought again, but how realistic is that? Better to be prepared, in case one of those thoughts pops up and threatens to trigger old and unhealthy habits.

Let's say you're filling in your calendar and realize that the beach BBQ for work is only two weeks away. Quickly you fall into old ways of thinking and talking to yourself, "What, two weeks!? I can't go to the party looking like this. If I really cut back and start going to the gym every day, I should be able to lose at least 10 pounds before the BBQ. I'm starting a diet first thing tomorrow morning."

The automatic thought, "People at the BBQ are going to judge me harshly for being so overweight," triggered anxiety, which in turn triggered a need for a solution. Presto, getting back on the diet merry-go-round is on your "to do" list again. Even if you know intellectually that dieting will only make your weight (and mood!) worse in the long run, the promise of a "diet that works" relieves some of your anxiety. And so, the cycle of weight loss, weight gain begins again.

Opposite action means that your behaviors don't have to be controlled by your thoughts and feelings. In other words, you can feel and think "A" and still do "B." So, if you think that you are going to be judged for your weight and that leaves you anxious, you still don't have to respond as you always have (for example, by going on a diet). Instead, you can take the *opposite action* in those situations, where your usual action will make your life worse in the long run. The BBQ will still leave you worried and anxious, but instead of doing what you've always done (begin another diet), you do the opposite (recommit to this never-diet-again program—a path to lasting weight management).

Here are some other examples that illustrate opposite action in use.

> **Action:** The day after a binge, you skip breakfast as a way of "making up" for the extra calories you had yesterday.
>
> **Opposite Action:** You make and eat a healthy, delicious breakfast. As a result, your blood sugar stabilizes more quickly and your urge to binge eat drops.

> **Action:** You eat more than planned at the company potluck. Now that you've "blown it," you decide to keep eating until you can't possibly fit in one more bite. After all, the day has already been ruined.
>
> **Opposite Action:** You still feel guilty and sad about overeating at the potluck. But instead of making things worse by launching into an all-out binge, you take a time out to recommit to mindful eating. By stepping out of the situation for a moment, you can reassure yourself that you are done with dieting forever, so there is no reason to "stock up" by bingeing your way through the potluck. If you eat any more at the gathering, it is because you are hungry or curious, not because you are anxious and frantic.

> **Action:** It's been a long week at work and you're overwhelmed and frustrated. You need a break from those feelings—and a big bowl of ice cream might just be the

quickest way to get that break. You're not hungry but you are desperate to not feel so stressed.

Opposite Action: You still feel overwhelmed and frustrated. Knowing that using ice cream to soothe those feelings will only work for an hour, tops, you don't binge on ice cream after all. Instead, you choose to do something that will provide more than temporary relief. Next thing you know, you're up to your chin in a hot bubble bath.

➢ **Action:** You're angry, angry, angry! Yelling at your boyfriend is the natural next step.

Opposite Action: You're still angry. But you know that you tend to overreact and have often (always, actually) regretted yelling at your boyfriend. It has never brought the two of you to a better place. Instead, you decide to talk to him with a particularly calm voice. Surprised, your boyfriend is far more willing to talk things through than he has ever been.

Wise Mind

Wise mind is when you think about things using both the logical side and the emotional side of your mind. Let's see how this might look in practice.

You've been invited to a wedding and dread showing up 30 pounds heavier than you were the last time you saw your extended family. Uncle Joe is sure to say something about you "packing it on" since the same time last year. If you let your emotions decide what to do next, you simply wouldn't go to the wedding. Your logical mind tells you that nothing earth-shattering will happen if you go to the wedding. People will say what they say and life will go on.

Wise mind, on the other hand, allows you to balance the logical and emotional side of the situation. Relying on your wise mind, you decide to go the wedding. After all, she is your favorite cousin. But, if the comments start to get to you, you have given yourself permission to take a time out. You'll take a walk outside or call a friend from the bathroom—whatever you need to do to comfort your emotional side.

The result is that logic and emotion equals a balanced approach to this situation. And this is key, your wise mind has allowed you to be effective—you've been able to go to the wedding, something you wanted to do, *and* take care of your emotions. Here are some other examples of wise mind at work.

> ➤ You've had a bad day of eating. From the morning through to the evening, you've been grazing. A handful of this, a handful of that. You're full (stuffed, actually) but still not satisfied. And, you are soooo frustrated! Why can't you get a handle on living a diet-free life without eating like a fiend? Your emotions are pushing you into two different, but extreme, directions. Either you're going to give up and let yourself gain and gain and gain, or you're going back on a strict diet in the hopes you will lose and lose and lose. The logical part of you knows that there are scientific reasons why dieting has never worked for you. The logical part of you also knows that giving up on your weight-management goals will harm your mind and body. So, what does your wise mind say?
>
> *Wise mind* integrates a (logical) commitment to follow a scientifically informed weight-management program (like this one) with a need to acknowledge that the slow-but-sure approach can be frustrating. You address the frustration by setting small mini-goals rather than

shooting for "complete recovery." Each time you meet a mini-goal, your frustration seems to fade a little bit more.

➤ You're madder than you've been in a long time. A colleague at work has taken credit for a project that you completed almost single-handedly. Logically, making a scene in the office is only going to get you into trouble. But emotionally, you're so angry, you're not sure you even care.

Wise mind to the rescue. You take the time to write your concerns and frustrations and run it by a friend to make sure you've managed to be firm yet professional. Off the letter goes to your colleague. And, you promise yourself, if it happens again, you'll take it higher. For now, you've communicated your concern (a logical first step) and used your anger to compose an assertive and compellingly argued letter to your colleague. Score two for you.

➤ Oh, yes, the gym. You're either on, driven by the logic that exercising is good, or off, driven by the shame and frustration you feel about your weight.

Wise mind is what leads you to sign up at a women's only gym and go when the gym is the least crowded. Sure, you could push through your emotions and force yourself to go when the gym is packed. But if you can go at a time that is easier on you emotionally, then wise mind tells you that you're being effective. You are getting the exercise you need while reducing your anxiety. Win-win.

Distraction

Sometimes you just need a break from all the worries, anxiety, and negative self-talk filling your head. For those of you who have yoyo dieted for years, you know all about taking a break by using food. The sleeve of cookies that keeps you company, and distracts you from the fight you had with your mother this morning, works for a good 15 minutes. But then you're back to the same old worries, only now you also have to deal with eating 20 cookies that you didn't even really like.

That's where preplanned, easy access *distraction* comes in. Breaks are good, you just need to make sure the breaks move you toward, not away from, your goals. Take the time to write a list of ways you can pass time without going overboard with the distraction (for example, four hours of video gaming is not where we are headed with this) and which really do boost your spirits. And make sure you include distractions you can do no matter where you are—if yoga helps you shift your focus away from "I hate my body" thoughts, but you can't pull out a mat in the middle of the office, then you need some work-friendly options. And, please, please, don't wait until you feel totally overwhelmed to practice your distractions. Try them on for size, even when you're having a good day—that way they'll be ready to go when you really need them. Want some suggestions? Here you are!

- ➢ Do something for someone else. It can be a random act of kindness, sending a postcard to a friend, or cleaning the car, even though it's not your turn.

- ➢ Pull out your favorite crafts—or try a new one on for size. You can even combine random act of kindness with crafts by knitting a hat for a preemie at your local hospital.

- ➢ Music, music, and more music. Listen to your favorite playlist or, even better, create one that only includes upbeat and encouraging music. Who hasn't had a day when they needed something like that?

- ➢ Count your blessings—literally. Make a numbered list of all the things you're grateful for—review it a few times.

Focusing on gratitude makes it harder to obsess about everything that is wrong in your life.

➢ Volunteer—Helping others, even for an hour or two a month, can really shift your perspective and help you realign your priorities. It can also get you out of your head and focused on giving to others, instead of dwelling on your own frustrations.

Just like the rest of this program, these skills really can work their weight-management magic if practiced and implemented when the time comes. But remember, not every skill works in every situation. It's kind of like a hammer. A hammer is a mighty handy tool but it isn't great for flipping pancakes or opening a can of peas. That's why it's a really good idea to also have a pancake turner and a can opener on hand. That same perspective is true for the skills that can help you master weight management once and for all. Make sure you don't only have a "hammer" in your tool box.

CHAPTER 19

Words of Wisdom When the Going Gets Tough

"Many of life's failures are people who did not realize how close they were to success when they gave up."

—THOMAS EDISON

When trying to break out of long-standing bad habits, chances are there will be times when you really could use a boost. This is particularly true if you've been working hard, but feel like you're not getting anywhere—or worse, like you're slipping backwards. For example, what if you're "working the program" and yet your weight is getting higher? The weight gain often reflects how slow your metabolism has become after years of dieting plus some natural "catch-up" eating that follows long-term dieting.

Still, it can be hard to keep that in mind when you feel bigger than ever. Suddenly you're at risk of reversing all your progress and retreating back to the "devil you know"—the same dieting that has triggered rebound weight gain over and over. This is just one of the times when inspiring quotes can give your Shattering the Yoyo journey its second wind. Here are some of my favorites.

You have power over your mind—not outside events.
Realize this, and you will find strength.
—MARCUS AURELIUS

You are imperfect, permanently and inevitably flawed.
And you are beautiful.
—AMY BLOOM

When you starve yourself, you feed your demons.
—UNKNOWN

In any given moment, we have two options: to step
forward into growth or to step back into safety.
—ABRAHAM MASLOW

They always say time changes things, but you actually
have to change them yourself.
—ANDY WARHOL

Believe you can and you're halfway there.
—THEODORE ROOSEVELT

He who controls others might be powerful, but he who
has mastered himself is mightier still.
—LAO TZU

Your body is precious. It is your vehicle for awakening.
Treat it with care.
—BUDDHA

I am beginning to measure myself in strength, not pounds. Sometimes in smiles.

—LAURIE HALSE ANDERSON

You, yourself, as much as anybody in the entire universe, deserve your love and affection.

—BUDDHA

Though no one can go back and make a brand new start, anyone can start from now and make a brand new ending.

—CARL BARD

Your mind will answer most questions if you learn to relax and wait for the answer.

—WILLIAM S. BURROUGHS

Nothing external to you has any power over you.

—RALPH WALDO EMERSON

Nourishing yourself in a way that helps you blossom in the direction you want to go is attainable, and you are worth the effort.

—DEBORAH DAY

Self-compassion is simply giving the same kindness to ourselves that we would give to others.

—CHRISTOPHER GERMER

Give your stress wings and let it fly away.

–TERRI GUILLEMETS

Sometimes the most important thing in a whole day is the rest we take between two deep breaths.

—ETTY HILLESUM

Make yourself a priority in your life. After all, it's your life.

—AKIROQ BROST

The most powerful relationship you will ever have is the relationship with yourself.

—STEVE MARABOLI

Love yourself first, and everything else falls in line. You really have to love yourself to get anything done in this world.

—LUCILLE BALL

To be beautiful means to be yourself. You don't need to be accepted by others. You need to accept yourself.

—THICH NHAT HANH

When you recover or discover something that nourishes your soul and brings joy, care enough about yourself to make room for it in your life.

–JEAN SHINODA BOLEN

Stop focusing on how stressed you are, and remember how blessed you are.

—UNKNOWN

Invent your world. Surround yourself with people, color, sounds, and work that nourish you.

—SARK (SUSAN ARIEL RAINBOW KENNEDY)

To love oneself is the beginning of a lifelong romance.

—OSCAR WILDE

Caring for myself is not self-indulgence, it is self-preservation.

—AUDRE LORDE

Learning to love yourself is like learning to walk— essential, life-changing, and the only way to stand tall.

—VIRONIKA TUGALEVA

Do something every day that is loving toward your body and gives you the opportunity to enjoy the sensations of your body.

—GOLDA PORETSKY

There's only one corner of the universe you can be certain of improving, and that's your own self.

—ALDOUS HUXLEY

Real change is difficult at the beginning. Without the familiar to rely upon, you may not [be] in as much command as you had once been. When things are not going your way, you will start doubting yourself. Stay positive, keep the faith, and keep moving forward— your breakthrough may be just around the corner.

—ROY T. BENNETT

We delight in the beauty of the butterfly, but rarely admit the changes it has gone through to achieve that beauty.

—MAYA ANGELOU

Just when the caterpillar thought the world was ending, he turned into a butterfly.

—PROVERB

If you're going through hell, keep going.

—WINSTON CHURCHILL

Develop success from failures. Discouragement and failure are two of the surest stepping stones to success.

—DALE CARNEGIE

Two roads diverged in a yellow wood . . . I took the one less traveled by, And that has made all the difference.

—ROBERT FROST

When one door of happiness closes, another opens; but often we look so long at the closed door that we do not see the one which has been opened for us.

—HELEN KELLER

When I let go of what I am, I become what I might be.

—LAO TZU

*Too many of us are not living our dreams because we
are living our fears.*

—LES BROWN

*If you do what you've always done, you'll get what
you've always gotten.*

—TONY ROBBINS

*When you stop chasing the wrong things, you give the
right things a chance to catch you.*

—LOLLY DASKAL

*Many of life's failures are people who did not realize
how close they were to success when they gave up.*

—THOMAS A. EDISON

*The thing with giving up is you never know. You never
know whether you could have done the job. And I'm
sick of not knowing about my life.*

—SOPHIE KINSELLA

*What you perceive as a failure today may actually be a
crucial step towards the success you seek. Never give up.*

—RICHELLE E. GOODRICH

*The definition of insanity is doing the same thing over
and over and expecting different results.*

—ATTRIBUTED TO ALBERT EINSTEIN

If we are to achieve results never before accomplished, we must expect to employ methods never before attempted.
—FRANCIS BACON

All changes, even the most longed for, have their melancholy; for what we leave behind us is a part of ourselves; we must die to one life before we can enter another.
—ANATOLE FRANCE

Any change, even a change for the better, is always accompanied by drawbacks and discomforts.
—ARNOLD BENNETT

When it becomes more difficult to suffer than to change . . . you will change.
—ROBERT ANTHONY

Take Action: Having read through this list of quotes, what did you connect with? What resonated with you? Pick out a few of your favorites and leave them in strategic places where they will motivate you! On your bathroom mirror, on your phone home screen, on your nightstand....wherever you think they may have value!

Trouble Shooting

CHAPTER 20

Getting Back on Track, When It Feels Like It's All Falling Apart

"What you perceive as a failure today may actually be a crucial step toward the success you seek. Never give up."

—RICHELLE E. GOODRICH

We have gone over what it's like to be trapped in the world of yoyo dieting. And we've gone over what it's like to leave that all behind by using new skills, challenging old thoughts, and breaking habits that haven't been serving you well. But what do you do if you seem to be going back and forth between the two? One day you're all gung ho, focused, and no longer letting automatic and negative thoughts control your eating. But the next day, you're knee deep in bags of chips, cookie crumbs, and despair. So now what?

This really is a good time to keep calm and carry on—in all seriousness. Recovery from the dieting/weight-gain yoyo isn't without some bumps and challenges. Falling back into old patterns is to be expected. It does *not* mean the program isn't working—it just means that, like a lot of people, breaking your habits sometimes includes two steps forward and one step back. The biggest risk when you are struggling to manage your weight, while giving up old patterns, is that you'll panic when the going gets tough and go back to dieting. It makes sense—it's what you know, and there is always the faint hope that, this time, restricting food will work. But, realistically, if it hasn't worked the past 50 times, chances aren't good that you're going to get what you're looking for from this week's "new and improved" diet.

Instead, use your energy to recommit to this program. Let it help you forge a new relationship with food, with your weight, and with yourself. But if panic about an episode of overeating is getting in the way of this commitment, here are a few things that might give you some relief.

1. Remind yourself why you decided to give up dieting. Maybe because it has taken up 5–10–15 years of your life with no lasting results. Maybe because counting calories has filled up so much of your brain's capacity that it hasn't left much room for anything else. Or maybe because you are tired of obsessing about your off-limits foods. Whatever it is, now is the time to remind yourself of all the costs of yoyo dieting.

2. Be kind to yourself—extremely kind! Another habit that can be hard to break is the shame, guilt, and punishment that can follow an episode of eating more than you planned, intended, or wanted. It's not uncommon for people to skip a meal (or meals) to make up for the extra food they had last night. But that only keeps the diet, binge, weight-gain, diet cycle in full swing. Try kindness instead. Treat yourself like you would a dear friend who was struggling. That might mean taking time to do something nice for yourself (a walk in the forest, a hot bath, reading a novel, doing your nails), asking a friend for support, or going out of the way to make your next meal particularly delicious and enjoyable. Whatever kindness is for you, you need to do it, instead of trying to berate yourself into making a positive change. (Doesn't work—millions have tried it!) Slips happen—perfection simply isn't part of this program.

3. When the dust has settled, take some time to understand what triggered the return to overeating. Were you overly hungry? Have you been getting enough sleep (honestly now, okay)? Are you overextended? Or, was it just an old habit coming into play, as sometimes happens. Whatever the triggers were, take some time to think about how you can respond to them differently next time. Maybe you need to keep a snack in your purse, so you don't end up famished after a long day of driving. Should you rein in the late-night YouTube watching or Facebook posting, so you can get the sleep you need? Or . . . well, you get the idea. Identify the situations that put you at risk of using food to calm yourself, and do your best to stay far, far away from them. In other words, review your danger zones, determine if there are any new ones that are catching you by surprise, and update your action plans.

4. Put biology on your side. If your slip was all about junk food (high sugar, high fat, high simple carbs), your regret and distress can unfortunately be accompanied by wonky blood sugar and feeling sluggish. Although no food is truly off-limits, when you are trying to get back on track, emphasizing protein, whole grains, and adequate hydration (water) is likely to leave you feeling a lot better physically than a couple of doughnuts washed down with a can of soda. That doesn't mean doughnuts or soda are banished from your diet, it just means there is a time and place for everything, and this isn't it.

5. Add to your "the things I've learned" list. As you go through this program, you will discover all sorts of things about yourself. Whether it is identifying the automatic thoughts that drive your yoyo dieting, coming to know the triggers that can send you back into old habits, or formulating the power thoughts that can keep you

headed in the right direction, you'll have learned a lot already. But it is easy to forget all the progress you have made when you're struggling. By keeping track of all the learning and progress that has happened, you will have a powerful tool at your fingertips. That's because reading it can keep the positives front and center. This makes it much harder for negative thinking to get in the way of sticking with the program.

One important point about managing slips is to make sure you are prepared well before they happen. It's like a fire drill—the point is to get you prepared to manage a fire when it really happens. Without that practice, you might find yourself running into a closet, rather than out the fire exit. So too with lapses, slips, or whatever you want to call it when your eating feels as if it has gotten out of control. You need to have a plan that you can follow automatically, rather than trying to come up with it in the middle of feeling panicky and desperate.

Take the time to fill out the form, "Things I Will Do to Get Back on Track using Kindness and Compassion," and list what you can do to gently nudge yourself in the direction of health when your eating hasn't been what you want it to be. Make yourself a "first aid" kit of soothing items (for example, candles, bath bombs, a favorite playlist, a foam roller . . . whatever you like) that are just waiting for you when you need them.

Have The Goals of Your Goals personal list, your "things I've learned" list, and your power thoughts ready and waiting at your fingertips when you need to give yourself a pep talk. The main thing is to make it as easy as possible to recapture your commitment to living a life free of yoyo dieting.

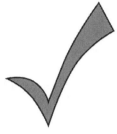

Take Action: So, it is going to happen—at least once, but probably several times. You are going to fall off track. What are you going to do to steady yourself and get yourself back on course? The time to decide that is now, not when you've already wavered. Think through your program and what you've connected with, and use the following worksheet to create your action plan for getting back on track!

Things I Will Do to Get Back on Track using Kindness and Compassion

THINGS I CAN DO TO GET BACK ON TRACK AFTER AN OVEREATING EPISODE
1.
2.
3.
4.
5.
6.
7.
8.
9.
10.

Case Study: Katherine and Bouncing Back

Does being kind to yourself really work? Well, let's take a look at Katherine's story. After 15 years of yoyo dieting, and a weight gain of about 50 pounds, Kathrine knew all too well the weight-gain/weight-loss yoyo. That's not to say she hasn't had moments when her weight dipped, and she felt like she was finally going to reach her goal. But it never happened. Inevitably she would "cheat" after ten days of dieting, then after seven days, then five, and finally it had gotten to the point where she only had a day or two of dieting in her before she would find herself gorging on ice cream or pizza or, usually, both.

After so many years of yoyo dieting, Katherine was at the point that it didn't take much to knock her off a diet. A little extra stress at work, a longer-than-usual commute home, or even a set of misplaced keys could send her running to the fridge. The next thing she knew, a half hour and about 3,000 calories had gone by. Then what?

Well, then would come the tears, the frustration, the guilt, and the regret. And usually there was some kind of plan to exercise the calories away and double down on her dieting efforts. That might mean skipping breakfast the next morning or adding 20 minutes to the treadmill work out that Katherine was already dreading. She hated every minute of hating herself for eating too much, of hating her body for being too big, and of feeling like she would never be "normal" when it came to eating and weight.

Sleep wouldn't come easy for her that night. Instead, Katherine would be left staring at the ceiling, wondering why it felt like she had the willpower of a flea and fighting the awful feeling that her weight wasn't going anywhere but up. But as much as

Katherine wanted to break this pattern, she didn't know there was an alternative to the false promises of chronic (yoyo) dieting.

Then came the Shatter the Yoyo program with its emphasis on self-compassion, changing old beliefs, and building herself up. And slowly things began to shift for Katherine. The first time Katherine felt herself slip into emotional eating, she also found herself falling back into scolding herself for being weak willed and a dieting failure. But, Katherine caught herself before these thoughts could trigger more dieting and exercise as punishment (rather than for enjoyment and health).

She took the time to remind herself that dieting hadn't worked for the past 15 years and really, there was no evidence that it would work in year 16. Katherine recognized that she would never tell her best friend to be ashamed of herself, or that she shouldn't eat breakfast after bingeing the night before. So, Katherine followed the slip, not with unkind words, but with her own homemade "spa" night at home—a bath, a home pedicure, and a facial mask.

Katherine was committed to giving herself the message that she was deserving, rather than the message that she needed to deprive herself. And you know what happened? The slips got shorter—partially because Katherine no longer needed to avoid the dieting that was just around the corner. She was able to do that because there was no dieting around the corner! Katherine's sadness about going back to old bingeing habits got lighter, and the time between her out-of-control eating episodes got longer.

CHAPTER 21

What to Do When You're Getting Better Slowly, But You Want to Lose Weight Fast

"Any change, even a change for the better, is always accompanied by drawbacks and discomforts."

—ARNOLD BENNETT

If yoyo dieting is so ineffective, why do people keep going back to it time and time again? As covered in the Introduction, dieting can be made to look easy and foolproof. How can anyone not lose weight on a program that is so neatly laid out and organized? Most of the time, people can lose the weight . . . in the short term. But the problem with the short term is just that, it's short. Most of our life takes place in the long term, and that's where rebound weight gain lives too.

Hopefully I've explained thoroughly to you why yoyo dieting is not the road to successful, sustained weight management. But what if you want (need?) to lose weight quickly. Maybe it's for a special event—a bridal party, a reunion, maybe even your own wedding. Or maybe you just can't stand to be in your own body. You want to be smaller, and you want to be smaller now!

You have officially arrived at an important fork in the road. One road leads to "weight loss now and weight gain later" and the other road leads to "Thank God, I'm finally off that soul-destroying yoyo dieting and letting my body let go of any extra weight at its own pace." Sure, an argument can be made for the "get thin quick" option—it's the same argument that fuels the diet-binge-diet-binge-collapse-in-despair-begin-again cycle. If you decide to go that route, just make sure that you are prepared to take the bad (weight regain) with the good ("lose 10 pounds in two weeks"). And keep in mind that the 10 pounds you "have" to lose this summer, might resurface as the 15 pounds you "have" to lose next summer.

Your approach to weight loss might start to feel, yet again, a lot like a hamster running on an orange plastic wheel—a whole lot of effort, without a lot of movement. For those of you who have a few more diets in you, the chance of winning the diet war might seem worth it. On the other hand, if you decide to be the turtle, rather than the hare, then keep your eye on the (right) prize. It's not short-term weight loss, and it's not a "bikini body" in time for summer two weeks away. It is the peace that comes with knowing that (a) you will never have to force yourself to diet again, and (b) you're slowly but surely moving toward your goal of arriving and staying at the healthy weight that is right for you.

Knowing that you are eventually going to be rewarded for taking the slow-and-sure approach to weight management is great, but what if your body image is so terrible that you can't think of much else? Is there anything you can do to make waiting for your reward less distressing? Truthfully, bad body image can be a tough nut to crack. Most everyone has messages about body, weight, and size that they've absorbed throughout the years.

These messages can leave you feeling inadequate and ashamed, when you feel like you've fallen short of the body you "should" have. And nowadays social media can make these feelings even worse by making us believe that "everyone" else out there already has that dream body! These negative feelings in turn leave you vulnerable to the siren call of dieting, and the next thing you know, you're back at square one, trying to lose the ten pounds you gained shortly after losing five.

It's probably not possible to make giving up the yoyo an entirely painless process. But it can be made more tolerable by putting a few of these tips into practice.

1. Don't let mirrors bring you down. Constantly checking your body size in the mirror can add to your distress. Sure, use the mirror to make sure you don't have spinach in your teeth or to work your mascara magic, but take a break from using a mirror to judge yourself again and again.

2. No tight clothes. Wearing clothes that are too tight can make it hard to think about something other than your weight. It's like when you have a pebble in your shoe, you spend all your time thinking about how much your foot hurts rather than where you're headed on your walk. Take a break from clothes you want to fit into "someday" and wear clothes that fit you (comfortably!) today.

3. Start thinking about your weight in a different way. Now would be a good time to practice changing your cognitive distortions into thoughts that build you up, rather than bring you down. If your weight has increased throughout the years due to the "side effect" of yoyo dieting, it is evidence that your metabolism, your appetite, and your fullness cues have been injured by your ineffective dieting efforts. It is not evidence that you're weak willed, a lost

cause, or a glutton. If you are carrying any extra weight, consider it a cast that developed in response to a dieting-induced injury to your body's weight-management abilities. Hold on to this thought, particularly when you're judging yourself for your present-day weight.

4. Focus on your authentic feelings of beauty. If you love your fingers, paint your nails beautifully. If your smile knocks it out of the park, let your teeth sparkle and your lips shine. If your hair is your calling card, treat yourself to a blow out or a deep conditioning in the comfort of your own home. The point is to find something, anything, that you can celebrate about your body and focus your attention there, rather than on the areas that keep you up at night.

5. Practice radical acceptance. There is a lot that can be said about radical acceptance, but for now all you need to know is that it is a technique that can help reduce the distress you feel in response to current realities. If you're the seventeenth person in the bank line on the Friday before the long weekend, then you're the seventeenth person in the line, whether you like it or not. You can be angry, frustrated, and impatient, but guess what? You're still the seventeenth person in the line. Or, you can accept that this is the situation that exists—no if, ands, or buts—and find a way to make the time pass as enjoyably as possible. Make conversation with the person next to you, send a friendly text to your sister, or hydrate yourself with the water bottle that you so wisely packed in your purse. Instead of using heaps of energy being frustrated, you can use it to make your life a little bit happier, friendlier, or healthier. That means if you're 250 pounds but really want to be 150 pounds, you can be angry, frustrated, and impatient (and 250 pounds), or you can shed the distress

and accept your weight as it is in this moment. You still weigh 250 pounds, but at least you're not making it worse with 100 pounds of negative emotions.

CHAPTER 22

A Body Image Gone Wrong . . . Then Radical Acceptance

"To be beautiful means to be yourself. You don't need to be accepted by others. You need to accept yourself."

—THICH NHAT HANH

Carissa hadn't always been concerned about her weight. She was a good athlete during her school years, right through until the end of college. Then came a desk job, weight gain, a diet after Christmas one year, and now, 10 years later, yoyo dieting and 40 more pounds. Carissa hated running into people who she knew from high school. Even if they didn't make any comments, she imagined what they were thinking. *How did she let herself go like that? Wasn't she the star basketball player from high school?*

But even worse than the real and imagined comments from others, was what Carissa said to herself. She'd catch a glimpse of herself in a mirror, a window, any reflective surface, and think *I'm so ugly. How did I get this way?!* These comments only added to Carissa's stress, which (thank you, cortisol) helped keep her appetite insatiable.

After 10 years, Carissa was finally and truly ready to break up with yoyo dieting for good. It wasn't an easy decision to make, because of how uncomfortable she felt in her body. But, eventually, Carissa was game to try anything, if it would give her a break from the voice in her head that just didn't shut up about her weight, her thighs, and her double chin.

Radical acceptance seemed like a bit (well, actually more than a bit) of a stretch at first. Carissa wondered if by "accepting" her weight as it was, she'd lose her motivation to make healthy changes to her diet and lifestyle. Instead, what she discovered was that the energy she had spent berating herself was suddenly available for other purposes. She used that energy to fill in the worksheets, take the steps outlined in this program, and to slowly but surely build a weight-management system that worked for her.

Radical acceptance didn't mean Carissa had to talk herself out of her body judgments, it just meant reframing her judgments as observations. It was no longer, "I'm 200 pounds. How pathetic!" Instead it was, "I'm 200 pounds. Period." Let's be clear, this wasn't an overnight process. But practice makes perfect. And after six months, the acceptance that at first seemed so foreign started to become a lot more automatic—and with it came a slow but steady downward shift in Carissa's weight.

SECTION 7

Putting It All Together

CHAPTER 23

A Week in the Life of a (Former) Yoyo Dieter, Before and After This Program

"In any given moment, we have two options: to step forward into growth or to step back into safety."

—ABRAHAM MASLOW

Part 1: Yoyo Dieting in Action

By the time Samantha made it to my office, she had spent more than 15 years (!) of her life obsessing about calories and exercise. She had also spent those 15-plus years losing and regaining (more) weight, so that she was significantly heavier than she had been when she first started dieting. She was, quite simply, dieting herself fat. After so many years of yoyo dieting, Samantha's self-esteem was really in the dumps. She felt completely inadequate compared to the naturally slim people in her life, who seemed to manage their weight effortlessly. She marveled at the fact that they could stop after two cookies, while she was lucky to stop after polishing off half a bag.

It wasn't for lack of trying that Samantha was getting bigger and bigger. She was constantly reading fitness and weight-loss books and magazines. She had filled journal after journal with food and exercise logs. She obsessed about calories, using any available head space to calculate how much she had to cut back to lose two pounds, each week for the next 10 weeks. To add insult to injury, Samantha was a health expert herself. Yep, that's right. She had a degree in public health, could talk for hours about the dos and don'ts of weight loss, and yet here she was, struggling ever day with her eating and weight.

The ripple effects of Samantha's dieting were vast. She isolated herself because she was so uncomfortable with her weight. She wouldn't even consider dating until she lost weight "once and for all," so she had been putting that off for years. There were so many hobbies Samantha would have loved to pursue—hiking, photography, travel—but it was all on hold until she finally found dieting success.

Yoyo dieting made it hard for Samantha to relax around food—she always felt like she was inches away from falling off the wagon and stuffing herself until she could barely move. Christmas was a nightmare for that reason. First, over the holidays Samantha would be anxious and irritable, as she tried to control her urges to eat all sorts of off-limits food. She would find herself daydreaming about mashed potatoes and stuffing and what it would be like to sit down with a big plate of warm apple pie and ice cream. Samantha would try to fight back with typical dieting advice—drinking so much water that she wouldn't have any room for "junk" food, eating a meal before she went to the party (not because she was hungry, but to leave her too full to eat any forbidden foods that might show up at the party), and filling up on vegetables (without dip) so that the mini-quiches didn't look quite so good. None of that worked. Samantha always eventually "blew it" and frantically binged her way through the holidays.

Of course, as a veteran yoyo dieter, that didn't stop Samantha from trying to diet for a day or two between binges, but even so, she'd inevitably end up pounds heavier by the time New Year's Day came around. Samantha had gotten to the point that she hated Christmas, weddings, Thanksgiving, birthday cakes at work . . . you name it, if it meant Samantha was surrounded by lots of good food, she hated it. Maybe being single was okay after all. She couldn't imagine trying to bring a husband and kids into this mix. (As true as that might have been, it was heartbreaking for Samantha, because she had always wanted her own family. Yoyo dieting was costing her more than she would have ever imagined!)

Part 2: This Program in Action

It took "hitting rock bottom" with her yoyo dieting on many, many occasions for Samantha to finally accept that dieting wasn't going to work for her. Maybe diets could work wonders for other people, but, for whatever reason, when it came to Samantha, another diet simply meant a lot of effort on her part without anything to show for it but weight gain. It was totally and completely crazy-making as far as Samantha was concerned.

That diets weren't going to work for her didn't change the fact that Samantha wanted to lose weight. The way she looked at it, it was yoyo dieting that had added the extra weight, not her genetics or "natural set point." If she was right (and she truly believed she was), Samantha didn't feel she should have to accept being a size that just didn't feel right to her. But, and this was a real breakthrough for Samantha, as much as she wanted to lose weight, Samantha wanted to stop obsessing about food even more.

This time Samantha was actually willing to stop focusing on losing weight and losing it fast, and was ready to do whatever she needed to do to be at peace with food. Once Samantha got to a place where thoughts of food weren't consuming nearly all her waking moments, well, then she would give some thought to what, if anything, she was going to do about the weight. Samantha didn't know what that might be, but she did know it wasn't going to be dieting. She'd fallen for that false promise one too many times.

When she began this program, Samantha had what I would call a honeymoon phase. She was confident, excited, and relieved to no longer feel that she had to count calories. This created a lot of momentum that Samantha used to identify the goals of her goals, to make time for self-care, and to start eating her off-limits foods. Samantha began with chocolate bars (a complete and total "no-no" on her yoyo diet, that she only ate when frantically bingeing after a "successful" diet), followed by French fries (which she really didn't like that much, as it turned out, but, after years of being off-limits, she indulged anyway), and then, ice cream bars—but not just any ice cream bars. Samantha went for the expensive bars with real chocolate coating.

At first, eating these foods wasn't as fun as it might sound. The calorie counting that she had done for years was automatic and extremely hard to turn off, on demand. It was hard to do, even though Samantha was giving herself permission to eat what she wanted. Panic would settle in as Samantha's calorie counting revealed numbers far higher than she felt she should be taking in on a single day.

This panic was joined by panic about weight gain. Although avoiding a scale like the plague, Samantha could feel her body getting bigger and her clothes getting tighter. And the truth was,

Samantha did gain a few pounds initially. That was predictable, given what she was eating. (Yes, post-diet, catch-up eating is a real, biological phenomenon!) This is where Samantha would have normally jumped right back on the diet bandwagon. It would have been all about reducing her panic in the short term by reining in her eating—even though rebound weight gain was waiting in the wings.

This time Samantha stuck to her guns. She began to challenge the "diet language" that permeated her automatic thoughts. *I have to go on a diet. I'm so out of control* became *I am choosing to relearn to eat normally. After so many years of dieting, it's only natural that I am eating a lot of my off-limits foods. But if I make them off-limits again, I'm back to square one. I need to give myself permission to eat these foods and eventually, they won't be so enticing.* Of course, this wasn't a one-time only conversation with herself. Samantha had to review her new thinking time and time again. Samantha made a top-10 list of power thoughts to keep herself going. "I deserve to have a happy and healthy relationship with food—and dieting never brought me that!" was said time and time again.

Samantha did a lot of work identifying her danger zones. She then made action plans so that she could get through those situations without eating everything in sight out of anxiety and habit. Yes, the random comments about her weight gain from "friends" and family were triggering for Samantha. Normally, they would have bought her a one-way ticket to binge eating. Instead, Samantha decided that every time someone made a comment, she was going to comfort herself with a nonfood reward.

After Steve at work commented that she looked like she had "packed on a few pounds" (Really, Steve? Why even say that?), Samantha took herself out for a fancy cup of tea at a high-end tea shop. It wasn't like Samantha to pay $7 for a cup of tea, but this time it was for a good cause. Samantha needed to know that she deserved kindness and comfort, even if (and maybe, particularly if) she had to contend with the food and weight police who sometimes seemed to populate her world.

Going too long without eating was another danger zone for Samantha. It used to be that she prided herself on her ability to delay eating while on a diet—she figured it was evidence of willpower, and, besides, it allowed her to "save" food for the end of the day—the time when she was the most tired and most in need of a break. But, more often than not, going too long without eating led Samantha to have such ravenous hunger, that the dinner and snack that was permitted on her diet wasn't enough to hold her. The grazing would start, followed by the convincing, albeit distorted, thought that she had blown it and might as well give up for the day. (Which dieters haven't talked themselves into "making a clean start" the next morning, all the while eating as much as possible in anticipation of the restriction to come?)

Participating in this program meant that Samantha knew that skipping a meal was just asking for trouble. It wasn't about willpower, it was about self-neglect. Samantha made a firm commitment to eat when she was hungry and always keep a few snacks with her, in case she found herself needing a nutrition break. Sure, it meant no more 4:00 p.m. lunches or 8:00 p.m. dinners for a while. But the stability that regular eating brought to Samantha (and her blood sugar) was worth it. She could eat dinner and move on to something other than food—reading, going for a walk, calling a friend. Compared to those nights when Samantha frantically ate her way through a box of crackers and a jar of peanut butter, those low-key activities felt a little like winning the lottery!

Samantha used a lot of other tools in this program to finally reach her goal of having a natural, stress-free relationship with food. Stress management, mindfulness, breaking bad habits and creating healthy ones, and providing herself with a nice environment to cook and eat were all part of the work Samantha did. It took a little more than a year for Samantha to feel "fully" recovered. Sure, it wasn't anywhere near a "lose weight fast" program, but the difference was that it worked and kept working. And, happily for Samantha, the longer she followed the program, the more her weight drifted back toward where it had been before her dieting took off in full swing. It drifted back, not because Samantha forced herself to cut back, count calories, or go to the gym for two hours, five times a week. It drifted back, because Samantha stopped being so interested in food when she finally stopped restricting it.

The reason this program didn't result in immediate weight loss was that it took Samantha's mind and body some time to truly believe that the next "no-fail" diet wasn't up on deck. Samantha's only regret? That she hadn't given up (yoyo) dieting earlier. Still, she chose to be grateful that this program had allowed her to take back her life—the life she had thought was lost to many more years of weight loss, weight gain, and food obsession.

CHAPTER 24

Next Steps

"Nourishing yourself in a way that helps you blossom in the direction you want to go is attainable, and you are worth the effort."

—DEBORAH DAY

My hope, at this point, is that you have made major changes in your life! You have truly changed your focus by reassessing your motivation, changing your outlook, and challenging old diet language. You have truly changed your thoughts by paying attention to the automatic, distorted views, and fighting back with your power thoughts. You have truly changed your life by changing your behaviors, including the bad habits associated with dieting. You've identified your danger zones and created and successfully implemented action plans that take all the danger out of these danger zones. So, now what?

Well, the hard part is done! If you have succeeded at everything in this book—you have done most of the heavy lifting! (If you haven't, you can revisit the chapters that you don't yet feel like you mastered, redo the worksheets, and continue to practice the included skills.) Now it's a matter of maintaining your success and directing it wherever you want to go. If you are happy with your changes and feel like they are moving you in a positive direction, then my only advice is be patient. As I've mentioned before, this is not a lose-weight-quick scheme. Slow and steady truly wins the race here. If you are making and maintaining all the changes outlined in this book, rest assured, they will have an impact!

If you want to continue the work you've started in this workbook, the next logical step is to enroll in my full online Shatter the Yoyo program. The program will review what was covered in this book, but it will also provide a substantial amount of new material. Some of these materials will cover other factors that can help further your ability to manage your weight successfully, sustainably, without resorting to extreme measures. As a preview to my full program, let's take a brief look at some of those factors.

Kitchen and Meal Time Setup

Believe it or not, the way you set up your kitchen and the way you plan and orchestrate your meal times has a big impact on your weight! Kitchen setup is one of those things that you don't really think about—you just do. For example, you just "know" that the veggies go down there, that you need this size of dishes, and that the toaster goes here. But those automatic thoughts are not necessarily what's best for you and often contribute to mindless eating and, eventually, weight gain! You need to identify these automatic thoughts, replace the distorted ones with healthier thoughts, and make some tweaks to your kitchen.

There are a lot of small changes you can make to the way you set up your kitchen that facilitate weight management and weight loss. In addition, the way in which you plan meals and set up your meal time can also have a hefty impact. In my full Shatter the Yoyo program, I walk you through all the kitchen and meal time factors that you need to pay attention to when trying to manage your weight. I will also help you create an implementation plan for the small changes that can result in big benefits to your health and quality of life.

The External Environment

Having read this book, you might be feeling like you are in good shape with all the content, have a lot more control, and a much better approach to behavior about eating. You have a plan and a system that set you up for healthy eating and good decision making. And all of this is wonderful . . . if you never leave the house!

The fact is that most people are equally, if not more, impacted by eating issues outside the house than they are by eating issues *inside* the house. These issues come at you from all directions! It might be a parent who's a food pusher. Or a restaurant with a mouthwatering image on the window. Or maybe the smell of fresh cinnamon rolls in the mall. Let's face it, a big chunk of the world "out there" is set up to make it incredibly easy for anyone to gain weight!

So, of course, you need a plan of attack—essentially a heavy-duty action plan—to be able to navigate the external environment without falling victim to the "eat, eat, and eat some more" message that is so pervasive. There are four main external environment areas and four useful ways to respond to each of these danger zones. In the full program, I discuss each danger zone and then help you formulate and *apply* the corresponding action plans.

Hunger and Fullness

It's hard to talk about food or eating behavior without talking about hunger. It's also hard to talk about hunger without thinking about fullness. The fact is that most dieters are completely disconnected from their hunger and fullness levels. So much so, that hunger is often not even the driver that makes them eat. It is often something else, such as the clock, a social event, or an emotional trigger. In addition, dieters are also often disconnected from their bodies' satiety signals—you know, that message that your brain and body send out when you're comfortably full. You've probably heard the adage that it takes 20 minutes for the brain to get the message that the stomach is full. What that means is that if your meal is going on and on, it's possible that whatever you've been eating for the past 20 minutes has pushed your body well beyond its satiation point. It might have been full 20 minutes ago!

Diets, by their nature, contribute to the disconnection from hunger and fullness signals. Thankfully, there is a way to reconnect with these signals, and there is a whole lot of benefit in doing so. One of the most obvious benefits is that it helps reduce overeating. It also allows you to create a healthier relationship with food, one in which you truly connect with your food and enjoy your eating experience. Being aware of your hunger and your satiety is also a major part of mindful eating, a topic that I will discuss shortly.

In the full Shatter the Yoyo program, I will walk you through the process of looking at how you can re-establish your connection with hunger and satiety. This ties into intuitive eating, an approach to eating that is critical to maintain a healthy relationship with food during the long term.

Mindful Eating

You have likely noticed many references to mindfulness throughout this book. That is because mindfulness is one of the most critical components to healthy eating behavior! When it comes to food, mindfulness is about being aware and connected to your eating behaviors. Many people are completely mindless when it comes to eating. Eating is something they do on autopilot or what they do while doing something else more important. Have you ever looked back on your day and had a hard time remembering what you ate? Have you ever wondered how you managed to eat the entire tub of popcorn without realizing it? Well, that's because your eating was far from mindful.

The problem with mindless eating is that it prevents you from connecting with your food—from truly appreciating and enjoying all the smells and flavors associated with it. It basically takes the enjoyment out of eating. I want to help you bring that enjoyment back!

I have worked with many, many people who claim to be extreme food lovers, but they eat so quickly that they barely have an opportunity to taste their food! Do you fall in this category? Loving food is about savoring it, and appreciating it with all your senses. Mindfulness is about getting you back to a place where you are present enough in the moment to do that.

The full Shatter the Yoyo program offers the opportunity to learn all the components of mindful eating. I will also introduce you to a system that will help you implement mindful eating practices into your everyday life. As with all parts of my full Shatter the Yoyo program, I don't want to just leave you with lots of information. I also want to make sure that you have ability to put the information into action.

Stress Management

It might not surprise you to see a section on stress management in a program about weight, right? As we reviewed earlier in this book, stress takes a major toll on your body and weight is a big part of that. If you didn't already know, you certainly know by now that stress can be a serious trigger for overeating. It can also make it hard to lose extra weight, in part due to cortisol, one of the hormones we met earlier. As a result, dealing with stress is a necessary part of dealing with your weight.

During the stress management modules, I will review both proactive and reactive approaches. Essentially, you can get in front of stress and try to *prevent* it from occurring, or you can try to *mitigate* stress once it's already happened. I will introduce you to stress-management strategies that you can use for both prevention and mitigation. As always, these skills will come with an implementation plan to make sure you use them effectively when the need arises.

Food Prep and Real Food

Food prep is an incredibly important part of my full program. You might notice I said *food* prep and not *meal* prep, and that was a deliberate distinction. For those of you on Instagram or other social media, you might be familiar with meal prep. You know, the pictures people post of 30 different pieces of Tupperware filled with premeasured and preweighed chicken, broccoli, egg whites, and avocado? I'm guessing you can already see that this doesn't exactly fit with the 80/20 mentality.

Every meal for the entire week is preplanned and selected and mostly allows for zero deviation—it's rigid, overcontrolled, all-or-nothing, and boring. (It also has a serious diet vibe going on!) Plus, what happens if something comes up and you can't have your preplanned meal, or, what if you just don't feel like eating it? Well, if the meal prep is part of an all-or-nothing, black-and-white approach to food, then you've just been set up for failure. When you have a plan that needs to be followed 100 percent, only following it even 99 percent of the time is a failure. You might just give up and go to the other extreme: "I'll just eat pizza the rest of the week and try again next Monday. Promise!"

This is the reason I purposely make the distinction between meal prep and food prep. I will be discussing food prep, because what I want to focus on is how to make good, healthy, and delicious options that are easily accessible. I will walk you through all the ins and outs of food prep and how to easily incorporate it into your work day/home life. I also provide lots of delicious recipes!

NEAT

There's a possibility you've heard people talking about NEAT and how to increase it, but you might not have any idea what it is! Well, NEAT stands for nonexercise activity thermogenesis. That probably still doesn't mean much to you! To put it simply, NEAT is really everything you do with your body, other than sleeping, eating, and exercising. Everything from cooking dinner to washing your face falls in this category.

Okay, so now you know what NEAT is, but why am I talking about it and what is it doing in a program on weight management? Well, the reason NEAT is relevant to this discussion is because the amount of thermogenesis (essentially, heat generation from burning calories) you have in your life can have a dramatic impact on weight loss and overall health. And, unfortunately, as technology improves, people are a lot less, well, thermogenic.

Imagine someone who gets up in the morning, drives to work, sits at a desk all day, hits up a drive-thru restaurant for dinner, and then spends the night on the couch watching TV. How much NEAT does that person have in their day? Not a heck of a lot! Now, imagine someone who gets up in the morning, walks the dog, bikes to work, works at a stand-up desk, cooks a nice dinner after work, takes a walk after dinner, and then straightens up the house. Now we're talking! That second person could be burning an additional 350 calories a day just from having more nonexercise activity! It doesn't take a genius to see how that can quickly add up to some serious weight loss (and some seriously enjoyable, productive, and mentally stimulating activities)!

NEAT is something you can easily incorporate into your daily routine without needing to find a lot of extra time. And, it has additional health benefits, such as reducing insulin sensitivity and diabetes risk, increasing strength and flexibility, and supporting posture and bone health. In my full Shatter the Yoyo program, I guide you through ways to incorporate NEAT into your daily life easily and enjoyably!

Conclusion

Food, eating, and managing our weight don't have to be so much work for so little payoff. When you finally decide that you are not willing to spend any more of your life going on and off diets, white knuckling it through potluck dinners, and avoiding the world because you are so uncomfortable with your weight, then you are ready to try something new.

This program can be that "something new" for you. And it can bring with it peace of mind about your weight, lasting success, and the satisfaction of knowing that you turned your back on the dieting that led you astray for so many years. This can be the beginning of a much happier, much healthier life. And if you want company on your journey to a life that is free of yoyo dieting, then my online program might be just the thing you're looking for. There is a private Facebook group accompanying the program to connect and gain support from others who are Shattering the Yoyo!

Not sure if the online program is right for you? Feel free to drop me a line at Info@TheWeightLossTherapist.com. I'd be happy to discuss your situation with you and determine if the program would be a good fit for you. In the meantime, I wish you all the best as you work toward freeing yourself from the yoyo diet trap once and for all.

Yours in Health and Happiness—

Candice Seti

Acknowledgements

There are so many people that have come together to make this book possible.

The editing and publishing of this book was financially made possible through a Kickstarter campaign. I would like to humbly express my immense gratitude towards all of my amazing friends, family, and other supporters that helped to successfully fund that campaign! A special shout-out to those that contributed WAY too much- Heather, Siwat, Paul, and Keith- you guys are my heroes and I love you to pieces!

I have been in private practice as a psychologist for many years now and have learned quite a bit from each and every one of my patients. All of my weight loss and weight management patients have contributed to the development of my program in one way or another. I would like to thank you all for your support, feedback, and commitment to me and the Shatter the Yoyo philosophy. I am so grateful for your dedication and I am so happy to see you all thriving!

I would like to thank Michele Hendsbee for being my first set of eyes on the original draft and helping me with expansion ideas. Your feedback was invaluable!

I would like to thank all of the copyeditors, artists, and publishers at Best Seller Publishing. I would have been lost without your direction and guidance! Thank you so much for helping me turn this into an actual book!

And finally, thank you to my husband Matt for the endless support. This book has taken up a huge chunk of my year and I truly appreciate all of your patience, understanding, and comfort!

About the Author

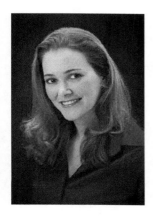

Dr. Candice Seti, aka The Weight Loss Therapist, is the world's leading eating and behavioral change specialist. She is a licensed clinical psychologist, a certified nutrition coach, a certified personal trainer, a certified weight management specialist, and a certified life coach. This unique set of specializations and education form the backbone of Dr. Seti's unique approach to weight loss and weight management.

Dr. Seti's approach is based on breaking dependence on diets and understanding our own thoughts and behaviors, so we can take control and end self-sabotage. Through this approach, Dr. Seti has created the Shatter the Yoyo program, which she utilizes in direct client care in her private practice. The program is also available online in a self-guided program.

Dr. Seti is also the author of the Binge Free for Life program, which utilizes a similar approach to help individuals change their relationship with food to ultimately break the binge-eating cycle permanently

Dr. Seti lives in San Diego, California, where she maintains a private practice.

Made in the USA
San Bernardino, CA
14 November 2017